DYING TO SAVE YOU

MW00526537

Dying to
SAVE YOU

And *Rebuild* Our
American Healthcare System

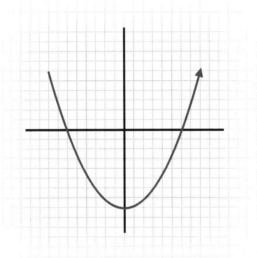

WILLIAM S. QUEALE, MD

LIONCREST
PUBLISHING

DYING TO SAVE YOU
And Rebuild Our American Healthcare System

FIRST EDITION

ISBN   978-1-5445-4155-6 *Hardcover*
       978-1-5445-4153-2 *Paperback*
       978-1-5445-4154-9 *Ebook*

To all those suffering from chronic dis-ease

Contents

Foreword

—GARY RICCIO, PHD

TRUST—IN GENERAL AND SPECIFICALLY IN HEALTHCARE—
is a two-way street that requires effective communication and
shared understanding. This can be extraordinarily difficult
when individuals have different kinds of expertise and communicate differently about their daily experiences. In this respect,
healthcare providers and their patients can sometimes seem to
inhabit different worlds.

The best way to overcome this impediment is through a
physician-patient relationship that develops across multiple
encounters over time. For this reason, Dr. Queale's book, *Dying
to Save You*, proposes that healthcare should once again be
focused on the relationship between patients and their physicians. At the same time, he acknowledges that this relationship
has become fractured due to inadequate time together and an
increasingly fragmented healthcare ecosystem.

Utilizing his extensive experience as a researcher, teacher, and clinician, Dr. Queale illuminates the forces shaping America's current healthcare system. He does this in a way that is neither esoteric nor ponderous. He writes in commonsense language that is rare, if not unprecedented, in expert opinions about healthcare writ large. As a result, his book will be revealing to healthcare providers and payers, as well as everyday Americans. He achieves this universality by adapting a time-honored tradition in medicine—clinical vignettes, or patient stories. Dr. Queale describes, often in exquisite detail, his encounters as a physician with his patients. Through these stories, he brings us face-to-face with human suffering, then he allows us to bear witness to lives being transformed through a process of healing. But in startling displays of authenticity, he also describes his own experiences as a patient struggling with the disease of addiction, and how his own life has been transformed through his experiences in recovery. This style, and the depth of relationships it conveys, is the most remarkable and, frankly, the most beautiful quality of the book.

While *Dying to Save You* focuses on the healthcare system in America, its guidance and implications are not limited to Americans and perhaps not even limited to healthcare. This is partly because it puts patients and providers on common ground, and that has value everywhere. It views a healthcare ecosystem beyond industry verticals, detailing the public and private economic systems through which healthcare is delivered. The book recognizes that, as economic systems, healthcare can optimize on whatever criteria it decides to organize around. Dr. Queale presents persuasive arguments that healthcare should be organized around a more inclusive set of criteria that address the whole person—an individual in the context of their own life. He also discusses how emerging science and technology could be applied to achieve these audacious goals, but only if primary care is given a more central role in our diverse healthcare ecosystem.

For those who are yearning for the promise of a better healthcare system, and for those who are seeking to develop it, Dr. Queale's book is a must-read.

Disclaimers

THE OPINIONS EXPRESSED IN *DYING TO SAVE YOU* ARE MY own. They are based on many years of education, training, and experience in many different healthcare fields and, more importantly, my experience recovering from the disease of addiction. The views expressed in this book do not represent those of any organization with which I am associated.

While I make suggestions in this book as to how a person can improve their health, this book does not constitute the practice of medicine, and no physician-patient relationship is formed. If you feel compelled to make changes to the way you live your life after reading this book, please seek the advice of a medical professional before doing so.

Finally, I tell many stories throughout this book. My personal story is my own and is true to the best of my recollection; after all, time has a way of shaping memories, and many were foggy to begin with. But I have made every effort to describe events in my life with the utmost accuracy in the hope that you might benefit from my experiences. The stories about my patients are also true; however, the details have been changed in different ways, often substantially, to make every effort to protect private health information. Some stories are composite cases, meaning that I have blended experiences with different patients to offer further anonymity yet still maintain the integrity of the message. Nonetheless, all of the stories in this book are based on actual events that I was privileged to witness. And I am grateful for the opportunity to do so.

Introduction

CHANGING TIDES

WHEN I WAS A BOY, I LOVED BUILDING SANDCASTLES ON the beach. They got to be pretty elaborate, with big walls and moats and towers. I knew the tide would come in and try to destroy my castle, so over the years I learned to build higher walls and deeper moats to keep the water at bay.

While playing this game with the incoming tide, I started to notice that low tide is calm and flat, quiet and simple. But high tide is more chaotic—the waves start getting bigger; there's more foam, more crashing, more energy, more turbulence. I could see the sand getting churned up and pulled out to sea along with little crabs and seaweed. Back to the ocean they went.

For the most part, I would sit in my chair behind my castle and watch it all unfold around me. Then as the big waves came crashing in, I would scurry around, reinforcing my walls and digging deeper moats to fend off the incoming tide. I got pretty good at defending my castles, but inevitably, the tide would always win. My sandcastle would always be destroyed.

Eventually, my family and I would leave for the day and go back to our beach house. The next day, I would walk back out to find beautiful, calm, flat sand. The tide may have washed away my sandcastle, but in its wake, it left a new foundation upon which I could *rebuild*.

Right there in front of me as a child, I witnessed a metaphor for the process of creation, destruction, and re-creation, which everything is subject to in this world. I didn't know it then, but this very simple yet profound experience would come back to me as I embarked on a journey through my own personal process of creation, destruction, and re-creation.

From getting into medical school to struggling with prescription drug addiction, nearly going bankrupt, and reinventing myself and my career, I have come to realize that everything goes through transformative cycles. And understanding these cycles might help us gain a better perspective of both human health and the entire healthcare industry. After all, both are in dire need of re-creation.

AMERICAN SICKCARE

Every day across the country, Americans are waking up to the same bleak reality: they are suffering from chronic disease and our American healthcare system can't save them. But, beyond chronic disease people are also experiencing *chronic dis-ease*—a general sense of uneasiness and despair that defies any actual diagnosis.

Perhaps you feel this way. I wouldn't be surprised. With the increasingly frenetic pace of society and a host of other environmental stressors, people's health is more vulnerable than ever. From severe storms ravaging coastal towns to new chemicals and plastics in our air, water, and food, from light pollution increasingly throwing off our circadian rhythms to vitriol spewed on social media, the cards seem stacked against us. On top of it all, the United States healthcare system has been failing us for decades, and many people have nowhere to go for help except the emergency room. It's no wonder people are losing hope in the future.

Undoubtedly, great advances have been made in human health in the past couple of centuries, with revolutionary drugs and surgical procedures increasing life expectancy. But we have also inherited a hobbled system of delivering and paying for healthcare, which has offset some of those great advances. This has left us in a precarious state: many people in the United States seek out, but do not get, the care they need.

Many don't even have a primary care doctor. If they do, they are often just put on drugs or punted from specialist to specialist, since the doctor has such little time to spend with them. Others simply cannot afford good care at all due to the staggering cost of good health insurance.

The effects are compounding: people are walking around with chronic physical and mental illness. Many will only get help after they cross some tipping point and have to be rushed to the hospital. But by then it's often too late because the damage has been done. These patients may go in and out of the hospital multiple times only to decline into a state of frailty from which they may never recover.

It's safe to say that we don't have a healthcare system in this country. We have a multitrillion dollar *sickcare* system, one that has come to depend on sick people to sustain itself.

Meanwhile, primary care doctors are trying to do what they were trained to do: keep people healthy and far away from this sickcare system. They want to prevent disease, or at least detect disease early and treat it before people end up in the hospital. So why aren't they?

One of the reasons patients lose out is because doctors lose out, too.

In the following pages, we will take a close look at how the system has forced primary care doctors to take on too many patients just to make ends meet, and how this increase in patient volume has led to increased physician burnout. Over-burdened primary care doctors have less time to focus on their own health. As a result, they run around in circles until they collapse and end up in their own emergency room. If they survive at all.

You can see the dominoes fall, can't you? How all the parts affect each other? We call it a healthcare *system* for a reason. Everything is connected. But like a patient with chronic disease, our healthcare system itself is sick. A system that might have worked well a hundred years ago is not working today in an environment of chronic disease—a theme we will revisit many times throughout this book. There have been many attempts to fix the system, but they have all been largely unsuccessful. Nothing we are doing seems to be working.

It's time to shake things up. We need a paradigm shift. We need a new approach to health and healthcare in America.

THINKING DIFFERENTLY

The foundation of medical science up to the present has been to drill down to the tiniest parts of a system and study those parts individually, as if they exist in a vacuum. This practice—known as *reductionism*—has been tremendously successful in generating new knowledge, leading to a progressively deeper understanding of human anatomy, physiology, cell biology, and genetics. On the other end of the science spectrum is *epidemiology*—the study of how diseases are distributed in large populations. Epidemiology has also led to great discoveries, including many public health interventions that have helped large numbers of people. But reductionism and epidemiology only help doctors so much when they have an individual patient sitting in front of them—a single whole person with a unique genetic makeup and set of life experiences.

Furthermore, physicians can't properly address all of the issues confronting patients if they only have fifteen minutes and a desk overflowing with administrative work. So the patient turns from a human being into a billing code; after all, the system deals with billing codes far better than human beings. But the person behind the billing code, with all their struggles, fears, and aspirations, is largely forgotten about, much to their detriment.

So how can we turn things around so that primary care doctors can attend to the actual *person* sitting in front of them? How can we get back to primary care doctors doing what they want to be doing: helping people improve their health and avoid disease in the first place?

The answer, as I see it, is twofold. First, we need a science that looks at the human body, its surrounding environment, and our medical industry as the *complex systems* they are—and we need technology, including artificial intelligence, to help us. Such a science would not only provide a more comprehensive understanding of human health, it would give us a new starting point from which to tackle the many political, financial, and cultural roadblocks to reforming healthcare delivery.

Second, we need to wed this systems-level understanding to a commitment to returning primary care to its rightful place as the entryway to healthcare—the interface between over 330 million Americans and a multitrillion dollar sickcare system. People are starved for access to a place they can go for comprehensive healthcare, a place where they will be heard and understood, treated as human beings, and given the attention and compassion they deserve. That place should be primary care. But right now our healthcare system isn't designed to pay for primary care; it is designed to pay for hospital care. And hospital care is what we are getting.

We need a reinvented primary care model that helps doctors build trusting relationships with their patients; provides care to all members of a community; focuses on the prevention, early detection, and treatment of disease with medical *and* lifestyle interventions; and coordinates care with specialists and hospitals when needed. A new primary care system based on this model could partner with our current hospital-based system to create a truly coordinated healthcare system—one that could not only reduce human suffering but also improve society as a whole.

Luckily, we don't have to invent this new way of thinking whole cloth. There is already a movement underway in America focused on applying the principles of systems science to the field of medicine. This science is using new data sources and computer modeling to understand how parts interact to form whole systems and how those systems adapt to changing environmental conditions. We will take a look at how these new technologies can be used to better understand human health and our entire healthcare system.

Having been in the trenches of primary care for over twenty years, I have seen everything—and I mean *everything*—at the ground level. But I have also seen the system at a high level as an advisor to large healthcare companies around the country. In fact, having these diverse experiences is how I came to write this book.

Three years ago, I was at a crossroads in my career and reached out to a good friend, bestselling author Joe Mechlinski, for some advice. After spending an hour listening to me unload my frustrations about our healthcare system and my thoughts about how we could improve it, Joe simply said to me, "Dude, you need to write a book." So here it is.

To help guide you, I have divided my book into three parts. *Part I: Our Healthcare Conundrum* focuses on the specific problems confronting healthcare, including why it's set up the way it is and why it's not working in the present day. These are the problems as I saw them with my own eyes—as a patient who was failed by the system, a physician who was almost bankrupted by the system, and an advisor trying to fix the system.

Part II: A Paradigm Shift focuses on how we can rethink key concepts in our present-day healthcare system. This includes how I came to believe in a systems approach to health and human disease; how experts are applying systems thinking to the field of medicine; and how you can take a systems approach to your own health and maybe avoid the sickcare system altogether.

Finally, *Part III: The Future of Medicine* focuses on how we can reinvent the primary care model and make it the foundation of a new American healthcare system. This system could not only reduce the burden of chronic disease and healthcare costs in this country but also improve society as a whole—if we make the right decisions going forward.

The current healthcare situation may be bleak, but I believe the future of healthcare in America is bright. True, I'm an eternal optimist. My own personal experiences battling addiction have taught me the power of community and fellowship. As a result, I've changed the trajectory of my life and my career to find solutions to my own problems.

But this book is not about me. It's about you and the millions of people who are suffering today just looking for some *hope*—hope for a better healthcare system and a new way of life.

PART I

Our Healthcare Conundrum

CHAPTER 1

Physician, Heal Thyself

AROUND 11:00 P.M. IN THE FALL OF 2001, I WAS SITTING alone at my desk in the basement of a little house in Baltimore City working on a statistical model for a friend. But it wasn't going very well. I had been up for about eighteen hours with the help of a drug called *Ritalin,* and I was exhausted just staring at the computer.

Ritalin, otherwise known as methylphenidate, is a *stimulant*—a drug that keeps you awake.[1] It is also a medication used to treat attention deficit disorder in kids. In my case, it was prescribed to combat severe *brain fog*—a feeling of overwhelming cognitive fatigue and mental slowness. The brain fog, my psychiatrist and I thought, was due to the side effects of the multiple antidepressants I had been taking for the deep, visceral pain of depression that developed during ten years of medical training. That's four years of medical school, three years of residency, and three years of fellowship, all on top of three years of graduate school and four years of college.

With seventeen years of education *after* high school under my belt, I thought I had checked all the boxes to get my dream job in academic medicine. My goal was to be a full-time faculty member and start a Division of Musculoskeletal Medicine. But things didn't work out as I had hoped. I didn't get the job. On top of that, my marriage was falling apart, and I was addicted to prescription drugs. Nothing, it seemed, was working.

Not sure what to do or where to go next, I just sat back and reflected on my life.

Little did I know it then, but that night was the beginning of an incredible journey of self-discovery. In time, this journey would not only lead me to reinvent myself, but also to wonder, *Could the same process that helped me rebuild my life also rebuild America's broken healthcare system?*

Understanding how I got to this moment will help you understand why the answer to that question is an unequivocal *yes*.

LIFE ON LIFE'S TERMS

I grew up a middle-class kid in a suburb northeast of Philadelphia. We didn't have much at the time, but we had enough to get by. In hindsight, we had more than many.

There were four of us in our family: my mom, dad, older brother, Bob, and me. My mom was a kindergarten teacher at a local public elementary school. My dad was a city planner. His job was to find common ground between private developers and local governments. Somehow he always seemed to find solutions that made both sides happy.

When I was young, my dad left his State job to start his own small consulting company. I watched him build his business over the years and would ask him questions about housing and other kinds of development. I'd also ask him what it was like to run a business. He would often say to me, "Bill, if you are good to your business, your business will be good to you." That sounded like good advice, but I would find out later on that it didn't apply to a doctor who was paid by an insurance company. We'll get to that later on.

In the meantime, school was difficult for me. I had a lot of trouble reading. I would often read a page ten times and still not remember what I had read. The fact that I wrote this book is ironic when you consider I almost didn't graduate high school because I couldn't pass my senior English composition class.

Plus, I couldn't pay attention to save my life. I was the kid who was always looking out the window, pondering the world around me, when a teacher would ask a question and snap me back to reality. I often felt stupid in school.

While I struggled to read, I loved to learn. This created a challenge: *I had to learn how to learn.*

As a kid, I dreamed about being an astronaut—after all, I grew up during NASA's Apollo and Space Shuttle programs—so I would always try to get my hands on anything related to astronomy and human spaceflight. Over the years, I taught myself how to scan books and extract information, but it was a tedious process, like mining for gold.

Learning, for me, was like going to school twice every day. First,

I had to learn what the teachers wanted me to learn *their way*; then, I would learn what I wanted to learn *my way*. Reorganizing information in a way that made sense to me was a skill I honed through practice over time.

Computers helped me as well. During the late 1970s, I watched firsthand as the computer industry came of age (these were the days of FORTRAN and punch cards). I had one of the first home computers, a TRS-80 Model 3 with a whopping 64k of RAM. My friend Tom and I figured out how to connect our computers over the phone line. We used to message each other over the computer rather than talk on the phone—somewhat like today's direct messaging. I also learned how to code, and soon I was writing my own programs to help me and other students study physics and chemistry. Little did I know that forty years later, it would be computers—and the algorithms they housed—that could underlie a new model of primary care.

Despite having a brain that never shut off, I was also physically active. Soccer was my main sport, but I dabbled in everything. I lived in a neighborhood with kids of all ages, and we did everything outside—flashlight tag, softball, kick the can, you name it. In addition, my friend's sister was dating a bodybuilder who would take us to his gym to lift weights. This was an old-school gym—straight out of the movie *Pumping Iron*. It was here that I would learn to lift weights properly and use nutrition to build muscle.

Unbeknownst to me, all these experiences I had as a kid were teaching me how physical, cognitive, and social activities impact our health and risk of disease.

TURNING THE PAGE

After negotiating with my high school English teacher, I did, in fact, graduate high school. I was looking forward to starting a new chapter in my life. I went to college at the University of Delaware to study physics, but I quickly turned my attention to biology and the human body. Since the days I started working out, I had always been fascinated by exercise and human performance, so I applied to the school's physical therapy program—and got accepted.

Studying the human body appealed to my intellectual strengths as a visual learner. I was able to get average grades in college without too much effort, which afforded me time to break out of my shell and have some fun. A lot of fun.

I spent my summers at the beach working as a bouncer and then a bartender. Talk about coming out of your shell. How I survived that much fun on those hot summer nights, I'll never know. But working as a bartender allowed me to see people for who they so often are—struggling humans. I've always said bartending trained me to be a better physician. It taught me more about human behavior, and humanity in general, than any course I could ever take in school.

After receiving my undergraduate degree in physical therapy, I stayed on to pursue a master's degree in exercise science. It was there that I learned how to push the human body to its limits. I also worked as a physical therapist and helped athletes heal from their sports injuries. I enjoyed recreational athletics myself—running, cycling, and strength training—and learned even more about how exercise and nutrition can improve human performance.

During graduate school, I also decided to challenge myself academically. I guess I was finally ready to get serious about my grades. For my electives, I took a number of high-level science courses—microbiology, immunology, organic chemistry, and biochemistry—and I did surprisingly well. Maybe *learning how to learn* was starting to pay off.

During graduate school, I also had the privilege of working part-time at The Johns Hopkins Hospital, where I fell in love with clinical medicine. I quickly knew it was my calling and decided I wanted to go to Hopkins for medical school. The problem? I had no path to get there. I was two years out of college with no premedical advisor or committee to help me.

I decided to seek the advice of a premedical advisor from another university. But after I told him about my academic career and my desire to go to Hopkins, he chuckled and said, "I wouldn't waste your time applying to Hopkins. You'll never get into a school like that."

I politely thanked him for his time and left his office.

As I walked to my car, I was pissed. I knew my undergraduate grades were pretty average, but the guy didn't have to laugh at the idea. I stopped and thought about it for a moment. Then I said to myself, *I am going to Hopkins for medical school. I just need to figure out how to get there.*

A BOLD MOVE

One day while working as a physical therapist at Hopkins, I decided to just walk into the Dean of Admissions' office for the medical school to figure out what I had to do to get into school there. The Dean wasn't available, but an affable older physician agreed to see me. He asked what he could do for me, and I told him I was interested in applying to their medical school.

"That's fabulous," he said. "What's the problem?"

"I was told not to bother applying here, that I'd never get in because of my poor undergraduate GPA."

"That's garbage," he replied. "We could fill an entire class of students with a 4.0 GPA if we wanted, but we like students with different backgrounds."

That was music to my ears.

"Of course, we need to know you won't fail the curriculum here," he continued. "That doesn't do anyone any good." Then he gave me the best advice anyone could give me. "Just do well on your MCATs. Often, a good MCAT score can offset an average GPA."

That was the answer I needed. The MCAT, or Medical College Admission Test, was my ticket to getting into Hopkins. I tucked that piece of advice away and went back to work.

That conversation set off a series of events that culminated in me applying to Hopkins as a "non-traditional" applicant. I studied my ass off for the MCATs and scored among the highest students in the country in all three sciences—biology, chemistry, and physics. My success in recreational athletics helped my application, along with my experience as a physical therapist and a bartender. But anyone who has applied to medical school knows the pain of waiting for a response.

Finally, I got a letter in the mail. I got an interview! It was one of 700 interviews out of 5,000 applicants, as I would later find out.

I did well in my interview. After all, what did I have to lose? But honestly, I think the interviewer was just perplexed by me. At one point, she asked, "Are you sure you want to do this? Do you know what you are getting yourself into?"

It was a fair question. I was making good money as a physical therapist and had a solid academic career in front of me, but none of that mattered. I felt medicine was my calling, and I had to pursue it. When I got my acceptance letter to Hopkins Medical School, it was an unbelievable affirmation that I had made the right decision.

In the summer of 1991, I moved to Baltimore, Maryland. I was twenty-five years old and in the best shape of my life. I thought I was invincible.

EXPLORING THE HUMAN BODY

Medical school was the epitome of *reductionism*—the science of breaking things down into smaller and smaller parts to understand how something works at the lowest level. We started at the top with gross anatomy. Dissecting the human body was a surreal experience—intellectual, spiritual, and creepy at the same time—but seeing the inside of a human body was a revelation. Every organ is different and unique. The liver, kidneys, heart, lungs—I could look at them with my own eyes and feel them with my own hands.

One level down, in histology class, we would look at these organs under a microscope. Magnified a thousand times, I could see groups of cells connected together—a small fraction of the billions of individual cells that make up one organ. And these are just a small fraction of the *trillions* of cells that make up our entire bodies.

I was fascinated by cells. They are massively complex and dynamic systems. Each cell in the human body is a small and bustling city in and of itself, all contained in a soft membrane like a water balloon. But cells do not live in isolation; they communicate with each other and work together in a coordinated fashion to form organs and tissues.

Inside cells, massive numbers of chemical reactions occur every second, allowing each cell to perform its specific job: nerve cells transmit electrical signals, liver cells metabolize toxins, immune cells fight off infections, and muscle cells keep us moving through our environment. Much of this activity is fueled by *mitochondria*—little power plants inside cells that convert the food we eat into energy to do work. Without well-functioning mitochondria, the body slows to a crawl.

At the lowest level is *DNA, or deoxyribonucleic acid*—a large molecule that contains the genes that code for little proteins called *enzymes*, which drive the chemical reactions. But genes are not static; they are turned on and off based on signals from the outside environment. The 1990s saw an explosion in technology that allowed us to sequence and even manipulate genes in the lab, and I jumped on the bandwagon. In 1992, I was accepted into a summer research fellowship at the National Institutes of Health, where I studied one part of one gene in one cell of the immune system. It was like studying one tiny piece of a puzzle with a trillion pieces!

I learned in medical school that we humans are remarkable creatures with the capacity to explore our own existence. And there I was, one out of 120 students at one of the greatest medical schools in the country doing exactly that. Ironically, the more I learned about the human body, the less attention I paid to my own. While I had entered medical school at peak physical and mental health, it was all downhill from there.

Like a car running past a red line, I was running myself into the ground. My body was starting to break down.

CASCADING FAILURE

My lifestyle changed dramatically during my four years in medical school. For one, I traded exercise for studying. As an early bird, I would get up at 3:30 most mornings during the week to study. The problem was, I often didn't get to bed until 11:00 p.m. or later. I was actually proud of myself that I could get by on such little sleep.

My diet changed, too. I ate what I could, when I could. Usually take-out food. Little sleep and poor diet—the first chinks in my armor began to appear.

My problems began compounding. I suffered from excruciating neck pain—an old college injury that had come back to haunt me. I even had to make a support for my head to relieve the pain while studying. To combat the stress of medical school, my friends and I would often go out for a few beers. Maybe more than a few on occasion.

During my second year of medical school, I got hit with viral meningitis complicated by a spinal fluid leak, followed by a battle with influenza. For someone who never got sick, there I was with back-to-back viral infections. What was going on? Perhaps I wasn't as invincible as I thought.

I was also dating a girl at the time, and during my second year of medical school, I proposed to her. Eight months later, we found out she was pregnant, so we got married and bought a small house in Baltimore City. Soon after that, I started developing pains in my stomach. They got bad enough that I went to see my university primary care physician, who put me through the usual battery of tests and said there was nothing wrong with me—that I was just anxious about getting married, having a child, and buying a house. So off to psychiatry I went.

That began an eight-year journey of psychotherapy, a slew of diagnoses, and more medications than I can remember. Meanwhile, I continued with my medical training. Balancing my personal responsibilities and medical care with my academic workload was a challenge, but I had never backed down from a challenge before. Why would I now?

Besides, I was beyond excited about being a father. When my little girl was born in August of my third year of medical school, I knew I had another calling besides being a physician: I was a father. That little girl was, and still is, everything to me.

I finished medical school and stayed at Hopkins for a three-year residency on the Osler Medical Service, named after the father of American medicine, Sir William Osler. The first year of residency is known as an internship. We were given as much responsibility as we could handle, routinely working over a hundred hours a week. It was not uncommon to work thirty-six hours straight. Sleep was a luxury, if it happened at all. That year was pure hell, but I learned a lot, and the friendships I made with fellow interns were lifesaving.

I was reasonably successful as an intern, since I loved caring for patients, but the responsibilities of the role didn't cater to my creative strengths. As interns, we were frequently required to do mundane work, such as drawing blood cultures, performing rectal exams, and giving stellar case presentations to your senior resident after not sleeping for twenty-four hours. Internship was beyond hard, and it started to take its toll on me.

At the end of my internship year, my wife and I had our second child, a little boy. Again, I was elated. After all, being a dad was my first job; being a doctor was second.

My little boy was born around the same time I had my internship exit interview, when my chief resident told me, among other things, something I would never forget: "Bill, you seem like an unhappy person."

Her statement caught me off guard. I loved being a physician, and I was at one of the best hospitals in the country. Plus, I had two beautiful children, a nice little home, four years of weekly psychotherapy, and a slew of antidepressants under my belt. Sure, I was in debt up to my ass, massively stressed, and chronically sleep-deprived. But unhappy? Clearly, something wasn't right. Over the next few years, I realized what she was talking about.

After my residency, I accepted a fellowship in General Internal Medicine at Hopkins. I wanted to be an academic physician—what's known as the *triple threat*: researcher, teacher, and clinician. Part of the fellowship included getting another master's degree, this time in epidemiology. The fellowship catered to my creativity and ability to multitask: I was a full-time student, saw patients in the student health center, covered the medical consult service, conducted my own research, and started my own primary care sports medicine clinic in the Department of Orthopedic Surgery.

To support my family, I moonlighted as an emergency physician and hospitalist in a local hospital. By this time, I had also become a team physician for the United States Soccer Federation and traveled internationally with many of our US National Teams. As if all these responsibilities weren't enough, I took on a role as team physician for Johns Hopkins University, worked with the NCAA to help redesign their Injury Surveillance System, and spoke at conferences around the country about a new field called sports epidemiology. To top it off, during all this chaos, I had my third child, another precious little girl.

TOTAL SYSTEM COLLAPSE

Perhaps not surprisingly, my fatigue worsened during those three years. Then the fatigue turned into pain—a deep, visceral pain that is hard to describe. The more I hurt, the more frustrated and anxious I became. I developed worsening stomach pains and recurrent bouts of lightheadedness. I also developed leg pain—a gnawing pain in both legs when I stood for long periods of time.

I sought help from my Hopkins colleagues, but my primary care doctor did not know what to do, so he sent me to a litany of specialists. An orthopedic doctor said there was nothing wrong with my back or legs but prescribed an anti-inflammatory drug. A gastroenterologist said I had acid reflux and prescribed an antacid drug. A cardiologist said my autonomic nervous system wasn't working and prescribed a medicine to control my heart rate. Everyone was focused on their organ system of interest, but no one, including me, was seeing the big picture.

While the medical doctors were all trying their drugs, my psychiatrist's list of possible diagnoses grew: depression, bipolar disorder, generalized anxiety disorder, and attention deficit disorder. The worse I felt, the more drugs I was prescribed. The more drugs I was prescribed, the worse I felt. Until one day, I was prescribed a drug called Ritalin.

Ritalin fixed everything—at least initially. It completely alleviated the massive fatigue and brain fog that overwhelmed me. Interestingly, it also cured my lightheadedness and leg pain. It seemed like the answer to my prayers. But unbeknownst to me, I was genetically susceptible to the disease of addiction. So when the drug stopped working, as usually happens with addictive drugs like Ritalin, I simply thought I needed more.

My psychiatrist was already prescribing the maximum dose and wouldn't give me more, so I just found a second psychiatrist.

Then a third. In my mind, I was simply doing what I had to do to keep going. But while I was able to maintain a high level of function on the outside, things were rapidly falling apart on the inside. I tried to stop the Ritalin on my own, but the pain and depression from withdrawal were devastating. I just couldn't function without that drug. I didn't know what to do.

By this time, it was about 2:00 a.m. on that early fall night. I sat down on the floor of my basement in a state of complete exhaustion and delirium. I thought to myself, *How the fuck did this happen to me? Where did I go wrong?* I felt completely defeated.

Then, suddenly, I started to tremble. Fear took over my body as if the devil himself had entered the room. My heart started beating out of my chest. I lay down on the ground and curled up in a ball. I remember thinking two thoughts as I lay helpless on the floor: *I can't take this pain anymore* and *My situation is hopeless.* I had put all my faith into our conventional medical system, and it was failing me. Where else was there to go? It was like checkmate. I felt like a wounded animal caught in a trap.

It was at that moment a horrifying thought occurred to me: *the only way to end my pain would be to end my life.*

REBUILDING

For anyone who has contemplated suicide, I feel your pain. Sometimes you get to the point where you just can't take it anymore. But suicide is a permanent solution to a temporary problem. As bad and hopeless as a situation may seem, I promise you, *it can get better.* Like a blade of grass growing through a crack in the sidewalk, human beings are resilient. We *can* recover.

I made a decision that night; I made a decision to press on through the pain and change the direction of my life. Shortly thereafter, I voluntarily admitted myself to an inpatient drug treatment center, where I was introduced to a program of recovery that I continue working to this day. Being with other struggling addicts meant everything to me. For the first time in a long time, I didn't feel alone. Little did I know that twenty years later, I would serve on the Board of Directors at that same treatment center.

I learned in rehab that healing would come not from adding more drugs but from *changing the way I lived my life*. First, I started working with my physician to develop a simpler and more individualized medication plan. After that, I started exercising again. Nothing crazy, just some light jogging and weightlifting. I had forgotten how exercise improved my overall sense of well-being. Then I started eating better. Not perfect, just better. And I slept! I had also forgotten what it was like to get a good night's sleep! Finally, I made the difficult decision to end my marriage. We gave it a good shot, but even my wife agreed it was time to move on. While that may not be the right decision for every couple, it was for us.

The hardest thing about getting divorced was not living with my kids full-time, but living a life of recovery has given me a relationship with my kids I never thought possible. It also gave me the opportunity to marry a woman who can only be described as my guardian angel. And with her came a beautiful stepdaughter, bringing our total number of kids to four.

Recovery has had one other profound effect on me. It has taught me to empathize with other struggling people. No, not everyone ends up in rehab and going to twelve-step meetings, but no one's life is perfect. *No one's.* Over time, I have also learned that the greater the adversity, the greater the opportunity for growth. And I use this knowledge every day to help my patients get through some very difficult times.

Is my life perfect? Far from it. Every day I struggle, and every day I fall short. But every day, I try to do better than the day before. Now here I am, over twenty years later, free from active addiction, having found a new way of life. So long as I follow that way, I have nothing to fear.

As it turns out, I'm far from alone in all of this. There are millions of people out there with worse problems and far less access to healthcare than me struggling to get help. And, like me, even if they seek out help, for a multitude of reasons that I will explore in this book, it's still an uphill battle to receive the care they need.

One of those was a patient of mine named Faith.

CHAPTER 2

Chronic Dis-Ease

IN THE FALL OF 2002, A PATIENT BY THE NAME OF FAITH
came to see me in my office. She was a high-functioning busi-
nesswoman in her forties, and she had been plagued by a series
of unexplained symptoms for most of her life. Only now they
were getting worse.

I learned in medical school that taking a careful history often
leads to the correct diagnosis. So, with an hour blocked off on
my schedule, I sat back, and we talked.

Faith told me she was well until the age of seventeen when
she developed *mononucleosis*—a viral infection common in
children and teenagers. Afterward, she started experiencing
severe, recurrent abdominal pain. None of the doctors she
saw could figure out what was wrong with her. At one point,
Faith was diagnosed with *Irritable Bowel Syndrome, or IBS*—a
collection of abdominal symptoms that defy a more specific
diagnosis. But she continued to look for answers.

"It's all in your head," one doctor told her. "You just need to relax, and everything will be fine." Sadly, that would not be the only time Faith heard those words.

As I continued listening to her story, Faith described how she got a bad insect bite at the age of thirty. A few days later, she became dizzy and couldn't sleep. Then she started experiencing relentless fatigue and brain fog. Her symptoms became so bad that they began to affect her work.

Faith sought help from another doctor. He couldn't find anything wrong with her either, so he diagnosed her with chronic fatigue syndrome. Like IBS, chronic fatigue syndrome is a nebulous diagnosis that doctors sometimes give when they can't figure out what, specifically, is wrong with a patient.

This diagnosis devastated Faith. In her competitive, fast-paced profession, chronic fatigue was the kiss of death. Worse, she couldn't tell anyone what she was going through. Not her colleagues, and certainly not her boss. If anyone found out about her condition, it could put her job in jeopardy.

Complicating Faith's situation was a contentious divorce that took a terrible emotional toll on her. With no help from doctors, her symptoms only worsened.

"I felt like I had been poisoned," she told me. "I didn't know what was wrong with me."

When she moved to a new state two years later, Faith thought that maybe a new home would bring better doctors and some help for her condition. By this time, she had started developing headaches—severe intermittent headaches for no apparent reason. Her new doctor diagnosed her with migraines and simply gave her pain medications. But while the medications helped her headaches, her fatigue went untreated and only grew worse.

By the time she got to me, Faith had suffered from low-grade fevers, swollen lymph nodes, and knee pain so debilitating that she had to slide down the stairs to get out the door for work in the morning. She was losing hope.

"Faith, I don't know what you have, but you have something," I told her.

Faith later told me those words changed her life. She said I was the first doctor who had made her feel like she had a real disease—who had validated her pain. That's how abandoned and hopeless the healthcare system had made her feel. If a doctor couldn't figure out what was wrong with her, she at least wanted to be taken seriously.

I ordered some blood work. The labs suggested an *autoimmune disease*—a condition where the immune system attacks the very body it's supposed to protect—so I sent Faith to a local rheumatologist. Unfortunately, the visit didn't go very well. After listening to her talk for a few minutes, the doctor stopped her mid-sentence and said, "Faith, I think I know what's wrong with you." She was so excited that a doctor finally had a diagnosis for her. She slowly leaned in to hear her diagnosis. "Your problem," he said, "is *stress*."

Faith didn't say a word. She just stood up and walked out.

Once again, she was made to feel like her symptoms were all in her head.

I was furious when Faith told me this story. I'll have a lot to say about stress in Chapter 6, but at that time, I needed a medical diagnosis. My gut told me something was seriously wrong, and I needed to know what it was.

Still suspicious of an autoimmune disease, I decided to try again, sending Faith to one of the best rheumatologists I knew at Hopkins. This doctor reviewed her records, listened to her story, examined her thoroughly, and said, shockingly, "Faith, my colleagues are idiots." It turned out Faith had, in fact, developed a severe autoimmune disease, and no other doctor saw it coming.

Faith was prescribed an immunosuppressive drug, and for her, it was a lifesaver. It was the first time she started getting control of her symptoms.

More importantly, Faith finally knew her symptoms were not all in her head.

AN EPIDEMIC OF CHRONIC DISEASE

Faith's story is not unique—Americans all across the country are getting crushed by chronic disease. According to the Centers for Disease Control and Prevention (CDC), chronic diseases are conditions that last one year or more and require ongoing medical attention or limit activities of daily living; they include conditions like diabetes, heart disease, cancer, dementia, and arthritis. Six out of ten adults in the United

States have at least one chronic disease, and four out of ten have two or more chronic diseases.[2]

But the numbers don't stop there. Chronic diseases are responsible for 7 out of 10 deaths in this country, killing more than 1.7 million Americans annually. They are also associated with significant disability. And the financial toll of chronic disease is staggering. Chronic diseases account for around 75 percent of all healthcare spending in the US annually. On top of that, they cost the US economy more than $1 trillion in lost productivity each year.[3]

If you add mental illness to the mix, the numbers only get worse. One out of five people in this country have some form of mental illness, such as depression, anxiety, and post-traumatic stress disorder; One in twenty have a serious mental health illness, such as major depression, bipolar disorder, and schizophrenia.[4] Worse, in 2020, 1.2 million people attempted suicide, and over 45,000 were successful.[5] That same year, more than 93,000 people died from a drug overdose, a number that increased to over 100,000 in 2021.[6] On top of that, about 140,000 people in the US die annually from excessive alcohol use.[7]

But even these numbers don't capture the *chronic dis-ease* that plagues many Americans on a daily basis—constant low-level fatigue, anxiety, and despair. For sure, chronic disease and mental illness cause chronic dis-ease, but there seems to be something else going on.

I recently had a patient say to me, "I'm not sure what's wrong with me—I just don't feel well." For reasons unclear to me, I am seeing more and more of these kinds of non-specific complaints in my practice. COVID-19 has certainly made things worse—especially the Long-COVID syndrome—but fear and rumors surrounding COVID-19 seem to spread faster than the virus itself. Add to that increasing political differences, global political tensions, economic uncertainty, and the vitriol spewed on social media, and it's a wonder we can function at all. Chronic dis-ease, it seems, is everywhere.

To make matters worse, our healthcare system isn't fixing the problem. In fact, it might be making it worse.

In reality, we don't even have a healthcare system in this country; as of 2021, we have a $4.3 trillion *sickcare system*[8]—a system that makes a lot of money off people being sick. While this system is good at treating acute injuries and illnesses, it is not very good at treating chronic disease. All our labs, X-rays, MRIs, CT scans, PET scans, and stress tests aren't providing all the answers, and all our drugs, vaccines, surgeries, radiation, and immune therapies aren't fixing all our problems. Even worse, the financial incentives of our high-volume sickcare system often undermine compassion and empathy. No one, it seems, has time to care anymore.

At a point when more and more people need more and more help, our massive sickcare system is leaving patients feeling frustrated, abandoned, and hopeless. Let's take a look at the absurdity of our problem. Perhaps some of this might sound familiar to you.

THE CHRONIC PUNT

Let's say you don't feel well. Maybe you are unusually tired and have some stomach pains. You call your primary care doctor for help, but the next available appointment is three weeks away.

When you actually go to the appointment, you sit in the waiting room and fill out a bunch of forms you've already filled out ten times before. Eventually you are brought back to a tiny exam room, where you put on a gown that doesn't fit and sit on crinkly paper that keeps sticking to you. A nurse comes in to take your vital signs, asks a few questions, then leaves.

Finally, a doctor comes in and you tell them about your problems. The doctor nods and taps things into the computer, not even looking at you, not even responding. You start to feel self-conscious and embarrassed because you suspect they aren't really listening to you. And they probably aren't! They are pretending to listen, but as we'll find out, the doctor's mind is on a million other things.

The long and short of it is that primary care doctors simply don't have time to listen to their patients. It's not that they don't want to—the system doesn't let them. They are often required to see twenty or more patients *every single day*! All they can think about is how to get a patient out of the office quickly. No wonder doctors only listen to their patients for about eleven seconds before they cut them off.[9]

Sadly, the system has forced primary care doctors to develop tactics to get you out of their office quickly so they can see the required number of patients each day. Let's take a look at a few of these tactics.

One way to get you out the door quickly is to simply order a bunch of tests. While tests can be helpful in making a diagnosis, they are often ordered without much thinking. It buys the doctor time, but it makes you wait another four weeks before another fifteen-minute visit.

Another way to get you out quickly is to punt you to a specialist. Don't get me wrong here, there are lots of good reasons to refer you to a specialist, but it's also an easy way to pass the buck down the line. It's one thing for a primary care doctor to be a quarterback of your care—it's another thing to simply be a traffic cop.

A more dramatic way to get you out of the office, or never see you in the first place, is to send you to the emergency room. As we'll see in Chapter 7, hospitals are great for life-threatening injuries and illnesses, but they are not so great for treating chronic disease. After waiting hours in the emergency room, you might get sent up to a hospital room, where overworked doctors and nurses do the best they can to provide high-quality, compassionate care. After a litany of tests, you often get discharged with no real answers, only to be sent back to the primary care doctor who sent you there in the first place. To make matters worse, you might get a bill from the hospital for services you never remember receiving. You could even be forced into bankruptcy. My friend Marty Makary wrote about this tragedy in his book *The Price We Pay*.[10]

But the quickest and easiest way for a doctor to get you out of their office is to prescribe a drug. Drugs are our favorite tools, and used wisely they can be lifesaving. But there's the saying: *if all you have is a hammer, then everything is a nail*. If that is the case, then our prescription pad is our hammer, and patients are our nails. But it works both ways. If you go to the doctor, aren't you expecting to be given a prescription? I mean, if you don't get a prescription, why even go to the doctor? You can take chicken noodle soup and Tylenol on your own.

The fact is, we love our drugs—doctors and patients alike. Our entire healthcare system is built around prescribing drugs. But sometimes, perhaps more than we want to admit, drugs can make things worse. I learned this lesson from a patient of mine named Melvin.

MAKING MATTERS WORSE

Melvin was an older man who had a slowly progressive cancer, along with multiple other chronic diseases. He was, shall we say, complicated. He experienced a lot of chronic physical pain, depression, poor energy, and decreased physical function.

I had prescribed my share of medications for Melvin, for sure, but he was also prescribed medications for various diseases by a number of specialists. He was easily on ten medications, but none of them seemed to be working very well. His cancer was progressing, and his pain and fatigue were just getting worse.

Because of his worsening symptoms, I referred Melvin to a *palliative care doctor*—a physician who specializes in relieving discomfort toward the end of someone's life. Of course this meant even more medicines. Some of the medicines made him nauseous, which caused him to lose weight. Then he got weak and had a hard time getting around his own home. Melvin was on a downward spiral.

One day, his wife called me and said, "Oh my God, I think my husband is dying." We immediately got him to the hospital.

I went in to see Melvin myself and remember thinking, *Holy cow, he looks terrible. He could die any minute.* The ER doctor agreed. None of us wanted him to die in the emergency room, so we all agreed to transfer him directly to *inpatient hospice*—a healthcare facility that specializes in helping people die with peace, comfort, and dignity.

One of the first things that happens in hospice care is that the patient is taken off all their medicines and only prescribed medicines for pain as needed. This is exactly what they did for Melvin.

Within a day off his medicines, he was feeling better. After a few days, he was sitting up in bed, talking to his family, smiling, and laughing. A month later, he was at his vacation home in Florida! Melvin was eventually put back on just one medicine to slow the progression of his cancer. He lived two more years before dying peacefully from his underlying disease.

It turns out, many of those other medicines that were supposed to be helping him were only making him worse. I had seen it many times before and even experienced it myself. But I had never seen anything quite like that before.

Unfortunately, our healthcare system is designed to encourage prescribing medicines and performing procedures. That's just how doctors, hospitals, and drug companies make money. Most doctors don't really like this way of doing things, but it's the system we work in.

There are many examples of problems caused by over-prescribing medications, but nothing compares to us causing the worst drug epidemic in our country's history.

THE OPIOID EPIDEMIC

In 1999, I was caught up in what would become the most extreme and tragic example of overprescribing this country has ever seen. I was a senior clinical fellow at Hopkins and wanted to start my own sports medicine practice. At the time, there were no non-operative orthopedic doctors, so I approached some colleagues and suggested I could help patients with orthopedic injuries that did not require surgery. Given my physical therapy, exercise science, and internal medicine training, I had a unique perspective on patients—I was able to see their injuries in a broader context. They agreed, and I started a first-of-its-kind, non-operative orthopedic sports medicine practice in the Department of Orthopedic Surgery.

Not surprisingly, a lot of patients who came into our clinic were experiencing pain. Anti-inflammatory medications and physical therapy were usually the course of action, but a new opioid drug had recently come out called OxyContin, which was touted as safe and non-addictive.

At the time, we were told not treating pain was not only unhealthy, it was not right. So every patient filled out a pain questionnaire, circling little sad and smiley faces to indicate their pain level. Pain, we were told, was now the "fifth vital sign" after temperature, blood pressure, heart rate, and respiratory rate, and we had to measure pain like we measured all the others.

I didn't like to see people in pain, and I certainly didn't want to be accused of being an immoral physician, so the prescriptions started flying. Knee pain? OxyContin. Back pain? OxyContin. Neck pain? Wrist pain? Shoulder pain? OxyContin. By the end of my fellowship, I was giving it out like candy under the assumption I was doing the right thing for my patients.

As a physician working in a local emergency room, I had the same pressure. In fact, every doctor in every hospital in the country felt this pressure. Either you treated your patient's pain with the new "perfectly safe" drug, or you were a bad doctor.

Fast-forward to 2007, when the Purdue Pharma lawsuit came out alleging Purdue was selling opioids through a deceptive marketing campaign that minimized their risks.[11] But by then, it was too late. The damage had been done. From 1999–2020, more than 564,000 people died from an overdose involving some type of opioid.[12]

Follow the science? Whose science should I follow? Purdue Pharma's science? I'll have a lot to say about science in the next chapter, but suffice it to say we physicians got duped and started a drug epidemic that has ruined the lives of so many people and their families in this country. Ironically, I would meet many of these people over the years in the rooms of many twelve-step meetings.

If it's not clear by now, many patients suffering from one or more chronic diseases have an uphill battle ahead of them when it comes to getting better. As we'll see, factors often beyond patients' control are constantly undermining their ability to remain healthy. And all too often, they blame themselves for their seeming failure to get a grip on their health.

There is no disease that better exemplifies all of this than obesity.

I CAN'T LOSE WEIGHT!

Gail, like so many people, was struggling to keep weight off. A career woman trying to balance work and raising a family, she was a classic yo-yo dieter—up and down and back up again. To make matters worse, she was on her way to developing diabetes, a condition that wreaked havoc in her family.

One day, Gail came into my office, and I noticed she seemed a little glum, unlike her usual upbeat self. I asked her about her family, kids, husband, and career. Then I did what I often do after I finish the more superficial part of the conversation—I looked at her and said, "And how's Gail doing?"

She just stared at me. Then the tears started flowing.

"I can't take it anymore!" Gail said. "I can't lose weight! I've put on thirty pounds over the past year. I don't know what's going on. I'm trying to diet, but the less I eat, the more weight I gain. I just can't do it. I hate myself and nothing's working!"

At this point, I put my pen down and we just talked. I needed to understand what was going on in her life. Why was she gaining weight? Why was her blood sugar starting to climb?

The thing about weight gain is that it's not just about eating. It's not just a calories in, calories out issue. When people have difficulty losing weight, it's more complicated than that. It's not as simple as saying, "Well, if you'd just eat less, you'd lose weight." It just doesn't work that way. In Gail's case, she was probably not getting enough calories, and along with some poor food choices, the wrong type of exercise, and high work stress, it was resulting in an inability to burn fat.

One thing I knew for certain was that the yo-yo dieting had to stop. We had to get back to some very sound nutritional principles, so I referred Gail to a registered dietician that I worked with. The main goal was to get her off sugar and processed foods and replace them with healthy foods, such as vegetables, whole grains, healthy fats, and adequate protein. We also talked about meal timing and not eating constantly throughout the day. By focusing on eating high-quality foods in a limited time frame throughout the day, we didn't actually have to worry about counting calories.

Next, I asked Gail about exercise. She did exercise occasionally, but it was high-intensity exercise early in the morning before breakfast. That's not always a bad program, but it was bad for her. When we perform high-intensity exercise in a fasted state, we often burn muscle for energy. And since muscle is where we burn most of our fat on a daily basis, the less muscle you have, the less fat you are able to burn. We talked about a number of different ways to exercise, and we settled on some simple brisk walking to conserve her muscle and improve her ability to burn fat for energy.

Finally, I asked Gail about work. It turned out she was on Zoom twelve hours a day for back-to-back calls using a small laptop. That's a long time to be on a laptop! First, I told her she had to go out and buy two large-screen monitors and a comfortable chair. This was to keep her from hunching over her computer. (Yes, changing computer monitors was part of the solution to helping her lose weight, since poor posture could cause pain and release stress hormones that can promote weight gain.) Next, she had to limit Zoom meetings to fifty minutes, not sixty; that would give her a ten-minute break between meetings. This was in addition to the half-hour break I told her was non-negotiable in the middle of the day. After dinner, no more work. Just rest and bed. You can't lose weight if you're not sleeping.

Over time, Gail lost the thirty pounds she gained and has since kept it off. More than that, she got her life back. As we'll see again later on, it wasn't costly pills or injections that helped her; Gail's weight loss was simply a byproduct of the new way she lived her life.

A COMPLEX SITUATION

Why do we have so much chronic disease in this country? Why is our current healthcare system failing so miserably? We'll spend much of Part II of this book exploring these questions, but suffice to say, Gail's difficulty losing weight wasn't that simple.

There were many factors affecting Gail's health, all of which were interacting with each other. Clearly, there were things Gail could do to help herself, and it was my job as her primary care doctor to figure out what those things were—but blaming herself for her weight gain was only making her feel worse. And that was making her more susceptible to bad habits.

Chronic diseases are not caused by being a bad person. We are all genetically predisposed to some kind of chronic disease, and the stress of society is only making things worse: we work two jobs just to pay the bills; we have new viruses appearing out of nowhere; news and social media convince us that our neighbor is our enemy. All of that makes us anxious, frustrated, or downright angry, driving cravings to relieve discomfort.

Of course, our food industry is right there to tempt us with snacks loaded with sugar and carbohydrates. If it's not food, it's some gadget pushed on social media that you really don't need. And, if all that fails, you can just go straight to alcohol or other drugs to feel better—there's no shortage of them in our society.

You can see how the chips are stacked against us, can't you? And yet, so many of my patients come in like Gail, hanging their heads in shame, on the verge of breaking down in tears because they can't get their chronic diseases under control.

Why is this happening? Why is the healthcare industry failing patients so miserably when it comes to preventing or managing chronic disease? To help answer this question, we need to understand what it looks like from the doctors' side. It turns out, it's not so great for them either.

CHAPTER 3

The Doctor's Dilemma

ONE EVENING AFTER A LONG DAY OF SEEING PATIENTS, I got a voice message from a woman named Jackie asking me to call her back. I knew Jackie well, having seen her during my fellowship days at Hopkins.

Over the phone, Jackie told me how she'd tripped on a sidewalk while out for a run. She landed on her elbow, and now her elbow hurt. But as I talked to her, something didn't seem right. Jackie didn't seem like herself.

"Did you hit your head?" I asked.

"No, I just tripped and fell. I landed on my elbow, and now my elbow hurts."

It was the end of a fourteen-hour day and I was tired, but I remember thinking, *I know this woman. There's something going on here.* I suggested she go to the ER to get an X-ray of her elbow and a CT scan of her head. But Jackie would have none of it.

"I'm okay. Let's just see how it feels tomorrow," she said.

I can only argue so much with my patients, so we waited until the morning.

The next morning, I saw Jackie in my office. Her exam was remarkably normal. I got an X-ray of her elbow, which was fine, but a CT scan of her head showed a tiny speck of blood in her brain.

I immediately called a neurosurgeon friend of mine, who arranged an emergency MRI and MR angiogram of Jackie's brain. It turned out she had an unusual *brain aneurysm*—a bulge in an artery in her brain—and it bled just enough to show up on the CT scan. We immediately admitted her to the hospital for emergency surgery, and after ten hours, her aneurysm was repaired. There was no more bleeding, and she was going to be fine.

Later, the surgeon called me.

"Bill, that was a great pickup," he said. "But I have to admit, I've never operated on this kind of aneurysm before. The only time we ever see it is on autopsy." Then he asked an interesting question. "What made you get a CT scan on this woman anyway? She didn't have any headache or neurologic symptoms, and her exam was normal."

"I don't know," I replied. "I know this woman. She's an athlete.

It didn't make sense that she called me just because she fell and hit her elbow. It seemed to me that something else was going on. Plus, I was worried about why she fell in the first place."

Did I get lucky? I don't know. *She* certainly got lucky. But it got me thinking: *If I didn't know Jackie as well as I did, I might have missed that diagnosis.* And that scared me. A lot.

Most doctors enter medical school excited, passionate, and idealistic. Then, we enter the real world—a world of massive debt, stifling bureaucracy, high workload, and fear of making a mistake and having someone die as a result. And if that weren't enough to worry about, we have to get the damn billing code correct.

THE CODING GAME

The Coding Game is exactly what it sounds like—a game we physicians play with insurance companies to get paid for our services. Here is how it goes: in order to get paid by an insurance company for a medical service, a doctor needs to submit a *medical claim*—a paper or electronic document that tells an insurance company what service was provided and for what reason. Every medical service is assigned a code, and every code is assigned a fee. Not surprisingly, this method of payment is called *fee-for-service.* In general, the more you do for a patient, the more you get paid.

Our current fee-for-service model encourages us to do more—more tests, more drugs, more biopsies, more injections, and more surgeries. There's always more a doctor can do for a patient. And, again, you wonder why we spend over $4 trillion every year on medical care in this country?

I never liked the Coding Game. Simply doing more is the wrong financial incentive for physicians; we should be incentivized to just do what is right for a patient, even if that is just listening. After all, I was trained to get to know my patients, ask my own questions, perform my own physical exams, and discuss my findings with my patients. I was trained to decide *with* my patient what next steps to take. None of this is very complicated, it just requires one thing: *time*.

Unfortunately, it turns out not all insurance companies value doctors spending time with their patients. It's just not the way the system is set up. This was a lesson I learned the hard way early in my career.

In the fall of 2001, I took over a small internal medicine practice outside Baltimore. The doctor before me participated in all major insurance companies, so I didn't have much of a choice but to play the Coding Game. Every patient in the practice was new to me, and I wanted to get to know all of them, so I made the commitment to spend one hour with every new patient. Eight patients a day, one hour per patient. Of course, there were add-on patients, phone calls, non-patient care work, and forms to fill out as well. Those were long days, but it was still nothing compared to what I had been through during my medical training.

After doing some homework, I figured out there were codes that allowed me to practice medicine the way I wanted. These codes weren't advertised, but they were out there, and they were legitimate. Some would allow me to deal with multiple issues in one visit; others actually allowed me to bill for extra time with patients. I practiced for two years using these codes, and most insurance companies paid them without question.

But toward the end of those two years, one insurance company owed me $85,000. It got to the point where I needed that money to pay my overhead, let alone take a salary. After hours of letters, phone calls, and phone conversations, they simply decided they weren't going to pay me. They denied all the codes I had submitted—the very codes I had taken from their codebook!

So there I was—stuck. By then, I was hundreds of thousands of dollars in debt between medical school and a business loan to start my practice. I was broke, financially and emotionally. I tried to shuffle some things around, but at the end of the day, things weren't working from a business standpoint. I was staring down the barrel of bankruptcy. Clearly, I had lost the Coding Game.

I reached out to a hospital billing expert I had befriended during fellowship to help me pull things together. She pointed out the problem pretty quickly.

"Bill, the problem is you spend too much time with your patients," she said. "If you want to stay in business, you have to see more patients—at least four patients an hour."

Four patients an hour is fifteen minutes per patient! There was no way I could see a patient every fifteen minutes! Not in primary care, anyway. Maybe when I was doing orthopedic work and seeing a patient for only one issue, such as knee pain. But in primary care, my patients often had ten or more active medical issues and were often on half a dozen medications. Not to mention they had complex lives that impacted their health. There was no way I was going to get through all that in fifteen minutes, let alone build a relationship with my patients.

At that point, I decided this whole primary care venture just wasn't working. If I couldn't take care of my patients the way I was trained to and the way patients deserved to be treated, then I was just going to get out of medicine altogether. *Maybe I'll start a landscaping company,* I thought. Anything to get far away from patient care at that point.

CREATING A NEW MODEL

I started making plans to get out of medicine and, yes, start a landscaping company. Then, one day I was talking to a patient about all of this. He was a businessman.

"Bill, you're a great doctor," he said. "Don't change the way you practice and definitely don't quit medicine. Just get out of insurance altogether and build a new primary care model."

I thought about it for a while. And that's what I did. That night I sat down and came up with a new practice model based on *quality* of care, not *quantity* of care. First, I determined how much time I wanted to spend with patients. Then I built in buffer time to take phone calls, add on patients the same day, check emails, and complete paperwork. When all was said and done, I came up with a number. I could take really good care of 300 patients—but no more.

The problem was, by that point, I had 1,500 patients in my practice. I wasn't even close to 300! I ran some more numbers. If I played the Coding Game according to their rules and saw patients every fifteen minutes, I could bring in about $300 per patient per year. Then it hit me. Instead of having 1,500 patients at $300 per year, maybe I could have 300 patients at

$1,500 per year. That would certainly allow me to provide good care to my patients.

Unfortunately, I knew insurance companies would never pay me that kind of money (even though they would benefit financially by me keeping my patients out of the hospital—more on that later). That meant I would have to charge my patients directly, and that meant a lot of patients wouldn't be able to see me. It was either that, or I quit medicine altogether.

Since I felt medicine was my calling, I really had no choice. I had to close my existing practice and start a new one based on this new model. It was a gut-wrenching decision, but that's what I did. I sent a heartfelt letter to my patients that explained everything I was struggling with, hoping they understood and that a small number of them would sign up.

Within a month, 200 patients joined my new practice. The ones that didn't sign up were overwhelmingly supportive of my decision.

The flak I got wasn't from my patients but, strikingly, from other doctors. Many thought I violated my oath as a physician and that I was just in it for the money. In reality, I wasn't looking to get rich off of my patients; I just wanted to spend more time with them and support my kids. This new model allowed me to do both—*practice better medicine and have a better life.*

This was all pretty new eighteen years ago, mind you. Today it's all the rage. The *concierge* or *direct primary care* model has gained acceptance in the private sector, and it might even be pressuring insurance companies to pay differently for primary care.

Unfortunately, the majority of primary care doctors still work under the same high-volume model we've had for decades. This is especially true in hospital-owned practices. Let's take a close look at a typical day in one of those practices to see the sheer absurdity of the hurdles they face.

THE DUMPING GROUND OF AMERICAN MEDICINE

When everything falls apart in medicine—whether it's a wound that gets infected or a prescription that was never filled—patients get dumped back to their primary care doctor. Now, we *should* be the primary point of contact in the healthcare system. But unfortunately, people often can't get in to see their primary care doctor because their doctor is overwhelmed with thousands of patients and mounds of paperwork.

The fact is, our primary care system is broken. It might have worked well a hundred years ago when things were more simple, but it is not working in an environment of chronic disease and complex administrative bureaucracy. What we have now is utter chaos.

Let me paint a picture for you. A primary care doctor's office gets calls from the moment they open to the moment they close and practically every moment in between. They have front desk staff charged with managing the barrage of phone calls and patients coming through the door. Then the doctors themselves are running around multiple rooms, plugging in unnecessary information into electronic medical record systems, and scheduling patients every fifteen minutes so they can make a living. Since up to a third of that fifteen minutes is used for paperwork, the doctors only have about ten minutes per patient face to face.[13] There's little time to even ask how the patient is feeling. Then there are the billing people, who are trying to play The Coding Game, and practice managers, who are trying to keep everybody organized. Finally, there are the medical records personnel who have to deal with a labyrinth of electronic medical records, since every practice and hospital has its own separate medical records system. Staff members might spend hours simply trying to track down records from other providers.

Electronic Medical Records (EMRs) are a whole other issue, one that could be a book unto itself. While there are benefits to EMRs in terms of administrative efficiencies and financial reporting, they have been wreaking havoc on physicians for the past fifteen years. Why? Because when physicians are required to use an EMR, their entire clinical workflow is disrupted. Everything they learned in medical school about how to care for patients goes out the window. Now they are just checking boxes in templates created by people who may have no experience actually treating patients.

Why are they using these medical record systems? Often because the hospital they work for requires them to use it. The sheer volume of medical claims now requires them to be submitted electronically. It's the only way to get paid. Not to mention all the billing codes need to match the diagnosis codes, and computers can do this easier than people. So, we're back to the Coding Game.

Then, aside from EMRs, there's the endless stream of prior-authorization forms. I've long lost track of how many times I've ordered a CT scan on a patient only to have an insurance company deny it. I need to order medicine? Denied. I need to get an MRI? Denied. I need to refer my patients to a specialist? Denied. We're constantly fighting with insurance companies. I've had situations where a prior-authorization leads to a phone call with a physician now working for an insurance company. I might be on hold for half an hour. I finally get on and have to justify my case. The whole process for just one prior-authorization could take up to an hour.

What if a patient gets admitted to the hospital? Now that's a nightmare. This is in part because primary care physicians are no longer involved in their patient's care. Patients are now cared for by *hospitalists*—physicians who specialize in hospital medicine. I don't disagree with the concept of hospitalists. In fact, some of my good friends are hospitalists. And given the sophistication of hospital medicine these days, having doctors specialize in hospital care makes good sense.

The problem is, hospitalists and primary care doctors are too busy to talk to one another. Neither one is at fault—everyone is just too busy. But often a patient's family calls me and says, "What's going on with my mother? They started her on new medicine and she's having an allergic reaction." I call the hospitalist, but they're in a procedure. I try to get information from the nurse, but they refuse to talk to me because of something called *HIPAA*—the Health Information Portability and Accountability Act. It is a law designed to protect patient privacy, but it has stifled communication between medical providers. So, we all play this game of trying to catch up with one another to communicate information to the patient's family members. In the end, no one is happy.

And that's assuming we can get our patients admitted to the hospital in the first place. It's not uncommon for patients to wait more than a day in the emergency room before getting admitted, but there is nothing we can do about it. The fact is, hospitals are overwhelmed with *potentially avoidable hospitalizations*—hospitalizations that could have been avoided because the condition could have been prevented or treated outside of a hospital setting.[14] Many people are there because they don't have a primary care doctor at all. They have no one to call but 911. This leaves little room for patients that truly require advanced medical care that only a hospital can provide. And COVID-19 only made the situation worse!

After discharge, the communication fiasco continues. Often patients leave the hospital and we don't even know about it. Then we're getting called by a home health company to sign a Medicare form so that they can get paid to provide home health care that we didn't order. Patients are also often discharged with new medications, so then we're calling in refills for medications we never started.

Simply put, medical providers often do not communicate with each other after a patient leaves the hospital.[15] Is it any real surprise that so many patients get sent back to the emergency room just days after they get home? Hospital readmissions are a major problem that is only made worse by a broken primary care system. We'll talk more about that in the next chapter.

And as if all these logistics aren't challenging enough, I haven't even gotten to the doctor's rulebook: *clinical practice guidelines.*

FOLLOW THE SCIENCE?

According to the Institute of Medicine (currently the National Academy of Medicine), clinical practice guidelines are "systematically developed statements to assist practitioner and patient decisions about appropriate health care for specific clinical circumstances."[16] In other words, they are the informal rules physicians are supposed to follow when making medical decisions. Want to order an MRI for back pain? Check the guideline. Want to prescribe a medicine for high cholesterol? Check the guideline. Want to prescribe a treatment for COVID-19? Check the guideline. Everything in medicine these days revolves around guidelines.

Don't get me wrong—guidelines are not bad. They can actually help physicians simplify complex problems. But they have changed the way we practice medicine.

For much of the twentieth century, physicians had to rely on the basic scientific knowledge and clinical skills they learned in medical school. The 1990s, however, witnessed the birth of *Evidence-Based Medicine*—a process to formally use research as the basis for medical decision-making.[17] And the primary science underlying Evidence-Based Medicine? *Epidemiology*— the study of how diseases are distributed in large populations.

I wanted to practice Evidence-Based Medicine, so during my general internal medicine fellowship, I pursued a master's degree in epidemiology at the Johns Hopkins School of Public Health. And of all the things I learned during my training, one thing stood out—it's really, really hard to conduct a good epidemiology study. Why? In part, because we are biased. All of us. We all have deep emotional attachments to what we believe to be true.

For example, are eggs good for you or bad for you? How about dairy? Red meat? Is a vegan diet more healthy? What about salt? Certainly salt is a killer. We can all agree on that, right?

Okay, forget all of them—let's go with smoking. We really do know smoking is bad for you. At least in the year 2023 we do, but in 1950, it wasn't so obvious. Maybe it was obvious to the tobacco companies, but they weren't talking.

We covered the opioid epidemic in the last chapter, so no need to discuss that again, but how about masks to prevent COVID-19? First we heard that masks don't work. There was no need to wear them, so we were told. Then, all we heard was that masks save lives—at least the lives of others, but they don't actually protect you. Then they said that masks might protect you, too, unless it's a cloth mask, and then it doesn't do anything. Then two masks are better than one. Finally, you don't need masks anymore, no need to wear them at all, at least if you are vaccinated. And are outdoors. Maybe. Now, again, they're saying masks do protect you. So wear one if it makes you feel better.

Everyone has an opinion on masks and data to back it up. The fact is, we pick and choose evidence to support our biases. We do it all the time. *All of us.*

Epidemiology is a great field, but to conduct an unbiased study takes time, money, and expertise. Take a typical drug study. Epidemiologists often use a method called the *Randomized Controlled Trial* or RCT to determine if a drug is effective. I'll spare you the details, but suffice it to say the RCT is the most advanced study design we have to minimize bias. But even a perfect RCT, one with no bias whatsoever, suffers from one major flaw—it only tells me about the *average* benefit of a drug in a large group of people. It does not tell me whether that drug will work for you as an *individual person.*

Let me walk you through an example of how this works. This gets a little in the weeds, but hang in there with me. It's important.

If I told you I had a drug that reduces your risk of dying from 20 percent to 10 percent over five years, it means it cuts your risk of dying in half during that time frame, right? Right. Drug companies would make billions of dollars off such a drug. If I told you I had a different drug that reduces your risk of dying from 0.2 percent to 0.1 percent over five years, that also cuts your risk of dying in half—another blockbuster drug! What's the difference? The difference is in the *absolute* risk of dying in the first place.

With the first drug, your *absolute* risk of dying starts at 20 percent and drops to 10 percent. That's a *difference* of 10 percent. That means, if I gave the drug to ten people, only one person would die instead of two. In other words, I have to give the drug to ten people to save one additional life over the five-year period. We call this the "Number Needed to Treat" or the NNT for short. For the first drug, the NNT would be ten. What about the second drug? It reduces the risk of dying from 0.2 percent to 0.1 percent. That's only a difference of 0.1 percent, giving an NNT of 1000. *That means I need to prescribe that drug to a thousand people to save one additional life!*

Now that's all very interesting, and maybe even a little frightening, but here is the more important point. With the second drug, how do I know if you are the one person in a thousand whose life will be saved? I don't. I have no idea. All I can do is prescribe it to a thousand people and hope for the best. Maybe that person is you. Or, more likely, you are one of the vast majority of patients who are prescribed a drug and it does nothing but potentially cause you side effects. As I said, epidemiology is complicated.

Clinical practice guidelines based on epidemiology are not bad. In fact, when they are done well, they can significantly improve clinical quality.[18] The key, however, is determining whether a specific treatment is right for a specific patient. To do that, we need to incorporate knowledge of a patient's genetics, biochemistry, physiology, and goals.

Unfortunately, we don't have accurate ways to collect all that information, nor do we have the science to understand how to put it all together. But as we'll see later on, this is exactly what a future primary care model could look like. In the meantime, we'll just have to follow the science as written in the guidelines and hope everything turns out okay.

But the dilemma faced by doctors is not just about which guideline to follow. As we will see, the cumulative stresses and strains on doctors from all angles are taking their toll. Sometimes, it can even be a matter of life or death.

DYING TO SAVE YOU

Physicians die from suicide at about twice the rate of the general population, with an average of one physician suicide every day.[19] But while the rate of suicide for male physicians is about

40–80 percent higher than the general population, depending on the study you refer to, the rate for female physicians is consistently more than 100 percent.[20]

Why would this be? What is it about practicing medicine that pushes physicians over the edge like this? It could have something to do with higher rates of depression and substance abuse, but it might also have something to do with conflicting job demands, an imbalance of work and family life, long working hours, and physician burnout.[21]

Physician burnout is a real problem. According to the American Academy of Family Practitioners, there is an epidemic of physician burnout characterized by physical, emotional, and spiritual exhaustion, compassion fatigue, and doubt about the meaning of one's work. It is also related to lower quality care, higher medical error rates, higher physician and staff turnover, alcohol and drug abuse, and suicide.[22]

The 2018 *Survey of America's Physicians* showed that 78 percent of primary care physicians sometimes, often, or always experience burnout. Furthermore, 62 percent are pessimistic about the future of medicine, 55 percent describe their morale as somewhat or very negative, 49 percent would not recommend medicine as a career for their children, and 46 percent plan to make a change in their career.[23] And that survey was before COVID-19!

The pandemic has only made things worse. Recent studies show that between 20 percent and 30 percent of all frontline healthcare workers say they are considering leaving their profession.[24] The numbers are even higher among primary care doctors. About 50 percent of internal medicine doctors and as many as 55 percent of family physicians reported they're seriously rethinking their careers or practices.[25] Whether this pans out is yet to be seen.[26]

I've known many doctors to leave the practice of medicine. Sometimes they go to work for insurance companies; other times it's a drug company, a biotech startup company, or the executive suite of a local hospital. The fact is, there are lots of avenues for doctors to make a living other than seeing patients, and many primary care physicians are taking advantage of the opportunity to do just that.

At the same time, the number of students going into primary care has been going down. According to a recent Kaiser survey, 2019 saw the lowest number of students entering primary care specialties on record. In fact, entry into primary care has been on the decline since 2011.[27]

This might, in part, be due to lower salaries. According to a 2019 survey, primary care physicians—defined as internal medicine, family practice, and pediatricians—ranked near the bottom of all specialties in terms of salary as the share of average revenue generated. They also had the three lowest salaries of all specialties listed.[28] With those kinds of numbers, it's no wonder fewer people are going into primary care. Who can blame them?

So if more doctors are leaving primary care and fewer are entering, who is going to see all their patients? Well, there's one terrible practice that's becoming more and more common— pushing the work onto nurse practitioners.

A NURSE PRACTITIONER'S NIGHTMARE

In the fall of 2018, I was attending a conference in Nashville when I sat down at my table and started chatting with the woman sitting next to me. Her name was Erin, and she was a *nurse practitioner (NP)*—a registered nurse who received advanced training to provide primary care services. It turned out she lived and worked only thirty minutes away from me! We hit it off immediately and I got to know her story.

Erin got her first job as a nurse practitioner in 2001, at a large primary care practice in Florida that was owned by a single physician. Her experience there was like baptism by fire. She had no orientation, she had four patients scheduled per hour, and on top of that, there were new patients added, with no limit to how many patients she could see in one day. It was total chaos.

"That experience really traumatized me," she said.

In 2002, Erin and her husband moved to Maryland, where she found a job in a local family practice that was owned by a group of physicians who had been friends since college and medical school. When she started her job, she saw two to three patients an hour. She worked closely with the physicians, asked questions, and updated them on their patients. She had a good working relationship with the doctors and enjoyed her job. But things were about to change.

In 2011, the practice was acquired by the local hospital. The entire staff, including the NPs, became employees of the hospital, while the physicians who'd started the practice remained as contractors. Then, a new physician was contracted by the hospital and joined the practice.

This physician didn't like NPs very much. In fact, when she started working there, she didn't like the small office assigned to her, so she kicked Erin out of her office and made her take the smaller one. Erin felt humiliated.

Then came the new electronic medical record system—or EMR.

"That was a nightmare," Erin said.

They had 17,000 patients in their practice, all of whom needed to be entered into the system. While the medical records staff would scan in old documents from their paper charts, they had to input all the pertinent medical data by hand. That was a huge task, and it wasn't easy. Figuring out where to input data in the EMR was impossible. They did the best they could, but patient care suffered.

A few years later, their local hospital was bought out by a large regional health system.

"That was like going from the frying pan into the fire," Erin told me.

That acquisition would bring a whole new set of changes to the small local hospital, including another EMR. Two physicians retired immediately. Then the pandemic hit and the support staff that was there to help with the EMR left because of the lockdowns. Erin and her colleagues were all on their own figuring out the new computer system while also trying to incorporate telemedicine, all with no support. They went to the hospital for help.

"I was in those meetings," she told me. "I would sit around a conference table and listen to the physicians complain about their need for more support. But I finally realized they had no say in how their practice operated once the health system took over."

Shortly thereafter, two more physicians submitted their letters of resignation. Then their long-time practice administrator retired. There were numerous other managerial changes and new titles for those roles. Erin didn't understand any of them, but she did know that morale was plummeting. There was no more sense of community at work.

Now the practice had only three to four people answering the phones, so patients were waiting on hold endlessly. They were told to use the patient portal on the EMR, but no one could figure out how to use it.

"I even had patients messaging me on social media because they couldn't get in touch with the office!" Erin said.

Trying to manage a full patient schedule, call back lab results, return emails, and manage telephone calls became unbearable. Erin did the best she could, but after nearly twenty years in family medicine, she couldn't take it anymore. So, there she was sitting at the same table as me in Nashville, Tennessee, looking for a new way to make a living.

After the pandemic subsided, I ended up hiring Erin. She's in a place now where she can develop a relationship with her patients and practice good medicine. But, sadly, not everyone is so lucky.

Erin's story illustrates a growing trend. As independent primary practices get bought out by local hospitals, and local hospitals get bought out by large regional health systems, primary care becomes more of a business than a profession. As doctors get more burnt out and their patient volume and administrative responsibility increase, they merely push their work onto nurse practitioners. Nurse practitioners are then left running from patient to patient, trying to fill the gaps and to make money for practices while delivering the best care possible.

It's a terrible solution to a terrible problem. It's not good for patients, it's not good for doctors, and it's certainly not good for nurse practitioners.

A NEW PERSPECTIVE

Our current healthcare model is one in which everyone loses. Patients lose because they struggle to get the care they need. Doctors and nurse practitioners lose because they don't have time to spend with their patients and are overloaded with administrative work. Ultimately, all of us footing the bill for high medical costs lose through high taxes and high insurance premiums.

By now, we might have an idea about the magnitude of the problem, but we still don't have any answers. We haven't even asked all the questions. To better understand the massive scale and sheer complexity of this problem, let alone how to solve it, we need a new perspective. We need to see our healthcare system from the top down, not just the bottom up. In 2011, in a twist of fate, I had the opportunity to do exactly that.

The next chapter is a little different than the past three. It tells my story as an adviser to a large healthcare organization and how I came to understand the evolution of our medical system over the past hundred years. To be perfectly honest, this can get a little monotonous. But as I learned in recovery, if we want a better future, we have to come to grips with our past. So let's move forward and dig in.

CHAPTER 4

The Payer Perspective

IN THE SUMMER OF 2011, SEVEN YEARS AFTER ESTABLISH-
ing my new primary care model, I headed to the Outer Banks
in North Carolina for a vacation with my family. Things were
going well, and I was looking forward to my next adventure.
Maybe it is time to grow my practice, I wondered. *Maybe I should
start a company to help other primary care providers transition to
this new practice model.* After all, this model saved my career.
Perhaps it could help other struggling physicians as well.

Little did I know the answer to my idle musings lay in my lug-
gage, in a new book that landed in my lap just before leaving
for vacation. But where did this book come from? And why
did it affect me so?

A few days before I left for vacation, a patient of mine came
in for a checkup. He was a *benefits consultant*—a person who
helps companies provide benefits to their employees—and
his specialty was health insurance. But he didn't just sell
insurance policies to these companies; his job was to help

companies become "self-insured." In other words, they cut out the middleman and basically *became the insurance company themselves.*

The day of his appointment, my patient gave me a book called *The Company that Solved Health Care* by John Torinus.[29] While I was on vacation, I cracked it open. Then, I couldn't put it down. It described the process of one company becoming self-insured and offering a new model of healthcare for its employees. This approach would not only save companies money, it would also help employees become healthy and more productive. And it instantly gave me a whole new perspective on our healthcare system.

While I had seen our system from the patient and provider sides, this book showed me the system from the *payer* side. In simple terms, a payer is anyone who is footing the bill for medical expenses. Often it's a private insurance company, but it could also be Medicare, Medicaid, the Veterans Administration, or now self-insured companies.

Seeing the system from the payer side gave me a thought. *Instead of fighting with each other, what if providers and payers joined forces?* After all, I knew my new practice model was working. Maybe we could tackle this healthcare problem together.

I got back from vacation excited to scale my practice model and partner with payers to reduce healthcare costs, but I didn't know which way to turn. Then, about a month later, by total coincidence, a new patient joined my practice who had recently been brought on as the CEO of a large national healthcare company. We both saw the opportunity to develop programs that could solve our healthcare problems at a national level, and I was hired as the company's senior medical advisor.

Being an advisor to a large national healthcare company helped me to see our healthcare industry as, well, an *industry*. I had seen it from the ground level as a doctor and a patient, but like Dorothy in *The Wizard of Oz*, I now got to see what was going on behind the curtain.

We have a complicated healthcare system, to say the least—a multitrillion dollar behemoth of an industry dominated by large hospital systems, pharmaceutical companies, medical equipment companies, and insurance companies. And this industry needs sick people to sustain itself. Worse, it's a convoluted, interconnected mess of public and private enterprises with all kinds of policy and business considerations. *How in the world do we even begin to fix it?*

I didn't have much experience with healthcare finance or policy. After all, I was a primary care doctor—a ground troop in our healthcare industry. So to tackle this question, I had to figure out how we got ourselves into this mess and the efforts taken to try to fix it.

Here is what I discovered.

HOW WE GOT HERE

A few hundred years ago, the transaction between doctors and patients was pretty simple. When a person got sick, they went to a doctor or some other type of healer, and with a bit of luck, they got better. They would pay the doctor somehow—often in trade rather than money.[30] But whatever it was, it was a simple transaction.

Things got complicated in the early part of the twentieth century. Science was evolving, and drugs like penicillin were discovered.[31] Surgery was starting to be performed under intravenous anesthesia.[32] And medical education was being transformed.[33] While hospitals had been around for nearly two hundred years, they started to expand to accommodate this new era of medicine.[34]

With hospital care came rising expenses. Some insurance plans began as early as the 1800s, covering specific medical issues like worker injuries. But it's safe to say that what we now know as modern health insurance didn't start until 1929 when Blue Cross, and subsequently Blue Shield, were created to pay for hospital and physician services, respectively.[35]

In general, the idea worked well. Patients who got sick could now receive hospital care and not worry about getting stuck with a large bill. But all of a sudden, we had what is now called a *third party payer*—an insurance company that collects money from you in premiums and then reimburses a doctor for providing services if you need them.

While all of this was done for the right reasons, it was effectively the beginning of the end of the physician-patient relationship. Before the involvement of insurance companies, the physician-patient relationship was sacred; doctors knew their patients, and patients knew their doctors. When insurance companies came along and started negotiating between these two, it was no longer clear who the physician's customer was. *Was it the patient? Or was it now the insurance company?* It appears to be both.

As healthcare costs continued to rise around the country, employers decided to offer health insurance as a benefit to attract employees. This is how most people got their health insurance over the course of the early to mid-twentieth century: it was offered and paid for by their employer, who bought it from one of these private insurance companies.[36] But what about the poor? The unemployed? The elderly and retirees?

Enter the federal government in the 1960s, which basically set up two programs: one was Medicare, a program that pays for medical care for seniors and people with disabilities, and the other was Medicaid, a state-run health insurance program for low-income individuals and children.[37] In theory, at least, everyone should now have some kind of insurance coverage with either private payers, the federal government, or state governments paying the medical bills. As we know, that's not quite how it worked out.

As science advanced, medicine followed. New medical procedures were developed, along with new diagnostic testing and medical devices. The pharmaceutical industry also exploded, offering lifesaving medicines but often at exorbitant prices—in part to recoup research and development expenses, in part to increase profits.[38]

At the same time, our modern lifestyle changed. The food industry changed, our environment changed, workplaces changed, and people started getting sicker. We started seeing diseases that we rarely saw before—chronic diseases like obesity, diabetes, high blood pressure, heart disease, and cancer. More disease meant more hospitals, more equipment, more suppliers, and more drugs. All this cost more money, which increased the demand for insurance.[39]

By the 1970s, a massive *medical-industrial complex* had emerged, composed of large hospital systems, nursing homes, pharmaceutical companies, medical equipment companies, and insurance companies.[40] It was also the beginning of a massive shift of wealth away from doctors and into the hands of these large corporations. Medicine was now big business, and as such, the cost of medical care skyrocketed—from $353 per person in 1970 to $12,914 per person in 2021.[41]

There were some early attempts at controlling medical costs, including the HMO industry that emerged in the 1970s. HMOs—or *Health Maintenance Organizations*—were top-down attempts by insurance companies to "manage" care and control costs. In this model, primary care doctors often worked directly for the insurance company and became known as *gatekeepers*—basically point guards navigating patient care—but this often led to restrictions about which specialists patients could see. And this lack of choice didn't sit well with people. The financial incentives were also reversed: the goal was to now provide as few services as possible to reduce costs—not the best incentive for good medical care.[42] Because of these and other issues, many HMOs fell out of favor by the mid-1990s.[43]

Then there were *Preferred Provider Organizations*, or PPOs—a model in which doctors in a particular area are included in the insurance company's "provider network."[44] I'm sure you've heard of PPOs or are even a member of one, but do you know how they control health costs? They have doctors sign contracts that require them to accept only the amount of money the insurance company decides to pay them.

As a result, and as I found out myself, doctors lose all leverage to negotiate their fees—or even get paid at all. As fees are reduced and practice expenses rise, the only way to stay in business is to see more patients, and that limits the amount of time doctors can spend with them, further eroding the physician-patient relationship.

VALUE-BASED CARE: GLIMMERS OF HOPE

By the turn of the twenty-first century, it seemed that incentivizing doctors to see a large number of patients might not be the best way to reduce medical costs, let alone improve patient care. As a result, policy makers started to focus on the *value* of care rather than the *volume* of care.[45] The concept of *value-based care* will become an important concept in Chapter 10, so let's spend a little time exploring this idea.

In medicine, value is defined as the health outcomes achieved per dollar spent.[46] To measure health outcomes in medicine, we use something called *quality measures*—numbers that represent something of interest such as medication errors or hospital infection rates.[47]

While I might not have used my epidemiology degree as an academic physician, I have used it a lot as a consultant, helping healthcare organizations improve the value of care they deliver to their patients. It didn't take long for me to realize, however, that measuring quality is complicated, and it often creates more work for the providers who are required to collect all the data.

After the Affordable Care Act was passed in 2010, the Center for Medicare and Medicaid Innovation (CMS Innovation Center) was formed to encourage providers and payers to get creative in building new models that emphasized the value of care over the volume of care.[48] For example, Medicare already had one program in place called *Medicare Advantage*—an arrangement where Medicare contracts with private insurance companies who pay for medical services to Medicare beneficiaries. Under these plans, the private insurance companies are incentivized to pay for high value services as a way to reduce costs. The more money they save in healthcare expenses, the more money they keep.

The most notable value-based care model has been the Accountable Care Organization, or ACO. ACOs are basically partnerships between *providers*—such as large physician groups or hospitals—and *payers*—such as Medicare or private insurance companies. Providers in ACOs are incentivized to work together and share data to deliver better care to their patients. If they are successful at helping payers reduce costs, they receive a share of the money saved.[49]

One of the ways ACOs save money is, no surprise here, by improving primary care! ACOs often use advanced primary care models—such as the Patient Centered Medical Home (PCMH), Comprehensive Primary Care Plus (CPC+), or Primary Care First (PCF) models—that all embrace commonsense solutions to primary care, such as improved access, better preventive services, and higher-quality chronic-disease management services.[50] And it appears these models work. In 2019, the Patient-Centered Primary Care Collaborative found that advanced primary care contributes to an ACO's success in improving quality and generating savings.[51] In 2020 alone, 67 percent of ACOs reduced costs for Medicare, saving them $1.9 billion.[52]

But while value-based care is the right direction and ACOs are good frameworks for delivering value-based services, they are not without their challenges. ACOs are large, complex organizational structures requiring a lot of upfront money and technology platforms to share data. Likewise, advanced primary care models can create a whole new level of complexity and administrative burden on primary care physicians. And this says nothing about how complicated and labor intensive it can be to measure quality and value. Still, despite these challenges, the spirit of value-based care is spot on: get payers and providers to work together to reduce healthcare costs and improve quality of care delivered to patients.

As a healthcare advisor, I have had a number of opportunities to help build out programs using value-based care models. Two programs stood out in particular because of their mission and success: one was designed to improve the health of low-income workers and the other to overcome socioeconomic barriers to care in disadvantaged communities. Let's take a look at each.

ON-SITE HEALTH CENTERS

When I started working as a healthcare advisor in 2011, I initially focused on self-insured companies. My CEO paired me with an operations specialist, and together, we learned everything we could about the problems faced by self-insured companies and the employees that worked for them. The experience was truly eye-opening.

One problem, no surprise here, was the prevalence of chronic disease. And while many companies had disease management programs, they were not helping much. Many disease management programs consisted of a nurse calling an employee at home to talk about their diet. Who wants to talk to a perfect stranger about their diet—let alone by telephone! Telephonic disease management programs run by insurance companies don't work very well. What works is having a meaningful relationship with a primary care provider who actually cares about you. We'll talk more about disease management in Chapter 9.

As we built out programs to deliver on-site primary care services to companies, another problem became clear to us. When an employee got injured on the job and did not get proper care, it often cost the company a lot of money. Although workers' compensation claims and medical claims are paid out of two different pots of money, they all affect the bottom line of a self-insured company.

One day, the company we worked for got a call from a manufacturing plant in Texas. They had a problem with high medical and workers' compensation claims and were wondering if we could help. We flew down to Texas to meet with the company's safety officer, who filled us in on their dilemma: while they offered health insurance to their employees, many were low-income workers who didn't have a primary care doctor to go to when they got sick or injured. So they would often go to the local hospital emergency room—even if it was just for a small cut! While the employee did receive medical care, it cost the company an arm and leg since emergency departments are expensive.

As we dug into the numbers, we found out the company was getting hammered in high workers' compensation claims, unnecessary ER visits, time off from work, short- and long-term disability, and high medical claims. At the end of the day, the employees did not have access to efficient medical care and it was costing the company a lot of money. It was a lose-lose situation.

After talking with the company's safety officer about how we could solve their problems, my partner and I decided to hire a nurse who was overseen by a local primary care doctor specializing in occupational health. This way, the nurse could treat a whole host of injuries and illnesses on site, and if needed, the employee could be seen by the primary care doctor in his office. If an injury or illness was more severe, care would be coordinated with a local specialist or hospital for proper treatment. The company loved our idea. We signed a contract and went to work.

The biggest challenge we had right off the bat was getting the right nurse. We knew employees would be skeptical of a nurse who worked for their employer. *Trust was critical.* We interviewed a number of qualified candidates and found one occupational health nurse who actually grew up in the town where the manufacturing plant was located. Many of the employees already knew her.

Once we got her on board, we launched a messaging campaign

to let all the employees know they had access to medical care on site. The employees loved it. On top of that, we built out programs to help manage workers' compensation claims. We also developed on-site injury prevention and disease management programs to keep employees healthy and free from acute injuries and illness in the first place. How did we do? Over the course of two years, our client saved over *three times* the amount of money we cost them for our services. More importantly, many low-income workers now had access to high-quality healthcare services for the first time ever.

What I learned from that experience was that value-based care works. When payers (a self-insured company, in this case) and primary care providers work together, they can improve the quality of care delivered to patients—and that actually *saves* payers money in the long run.

As we will see next, it's not only companies and their employees that benefit by working together—disadvantaged communities can benefit as well.

SOCIAL DETERMINANTS OF HEALTH

While we were getting our corporate health business going, a new federal policy went into effect nationwide. Under this policy, hospitals would be penalized if they had a patient readmitted to the hospital within thirty days of discharge.[53] This *hospital readmission rate* became one of the hottest quality measures in medicine. Every hospital in the country was going to live or die by their thirty-day readmission rate.

A few years after this policy went into effect, I got a call from my CEO. A local hospital administrator had contacted him to see if we could assist with reducing his hospital readmission rate, and he wanted to know if I could help. I told him, "Absolutely, I'm a primary care doctor, that's my job—keeping people out of the hospital!" He asked my operations partner and me to bat around some ideas and get back to him.

By pure coincidence, my oldest daughter, Julia, was returning from India at this time, after completing a nine-month internship with a non-government organization (NGO) called the Comprehensive Rural Health Project (CRHP). On our way home from Dulles International Airport, she explained to me the basic mission of CRHP: to provide equitable, community-based primary healthcare in villages around a town called Jamkhed, one of the poorest areas in Maharashtra State. Providing care to local villages, however, was not without its challenges. The rural location and impoverished conditions of the villages made the delivery of even basic medical care challenging.

But there was an even deeper challenge to deal with. The *caste system*—a hierarchical system of social and economic status—often left the poorest of the poor in these villages without access to any care at all. This marginalized group, called the *Dalits*, were mostly women and they were often disregarded by society altogether. In order to bring preventive and basic medical care to all members of the village, CRHP would have to tackle the inequities of the caste system.

In their book, *Jamkhed*, Drs. Raj and Mabelle Arole describe how they solved both of these problems.[54] They recruited and trained local villagers to serve as *Village Health Workers*

(VHWs). The VHWs would provide health education and basic health services, such as oral rehydration, first aid, basic medications, and even delivering babies. If more advanced medical care was needed, they would be taken to the hospital on the CRHP campus.

The VHW model improved healthcare delivery to the villagers. But what about the health equity problem? How did they ensure access to care among all villagers? Well, CRHP didn't just recruit anyone to be a VHW. *They recruited the Dalits themselves!* Doing so required the villagers to break their view of the caste system in order to receive the medical care they needed. It was a brilliant solution that allowed the poorest of the poor to receive equitable medical care, reducing the need for everyone to use the hospital in the city. More importantly, it brought the Dalits the respect they deserved.

I told my partner about my conversation with my daughter, and we immediately knew what we had to do. We had to solve the health equity problem in communities surrounding our hospital client.

We knew primary care doctors wanted to help, but there's only so much they could do in the office—especially with only 15 minutes per patient. If we wanted to help the hospital reduce readmissions, we had to help their primary care providers deliver care outside the office and *in the communities they served.* We needed to focus on the social, cultural, and economic barriers that prevented patients from receiving preventive and basic medical care in the first place.

We designed our own version of the Jamkhed model for our

hospital client, hiring a nurse practitioner to help us. Having grown up in Eastern Europe under the grip of the Soviet Union, she knew firsthand what it was like for patients to have difficulty getting access to appropriate medical care. Plus, having worked for an American insurance company, she knew how broken and fragmented the system was. Together, we built out a team and created what we called a Community-Based Care Management (CBCM) program.

As part of our program, we worked with a technology partner to identify hospitalized patients at high risk for readmission based on medical *and* socioeconomic factors. Then we hired people from different communities around Baltimore and trained them to be Community Health Workers (CHWs). Our CHWs were not medical providers; they were high school graduates, moms, dads, young, old—basically anyone who wanted a good, decent-paying job to help identify barriers patients had to receiving good medical care.

After a patient was discharged from the hospital, we sent a CHW out to their home to look for any reason they might get readmitted. The problems we uncovered were staggering. It turned out many people didn't even have basic resources such as food, safe housing, or transportation—let alone a primary care doctor. Sometimes patients had six or eight people living in one small house with no heat. Other times their children were taking what little money they had for drugs—leaving them with no money to pay for medications. Diseases like hypertension, asthma, heart failure, and depression went untreated until they led to an acute injury or illness requiring hospitalization.

No wonder they were calling 911 all the time. Once the *real* problems underlying readmission to the hospital were identified, our community health workers went to work. They did whatever they needed to get resources to their patients.

One memorable example concerned a woman who kept going to the ER for back pain. When one of our community healthcare workers went out to check on her, she immediately identified the problem: the woman didn't have a mattress to sleep on. She was sleeping on a hardwood floor!

To solve the problem, our community health worker went over to a local mattress store and asked them if they had any extra mattresses they were getting rid of. It just so happened they had some brand new mattresses they didn't want still sealed in plastic in the dumpster behind the store. So our community healthcare worker went to the dumpster, pulled out a brand new mattress, tied it to the roof of her car, and took it to this woman's house. Now the woman had a comfortable place to sleep and didn't end up in the ER for back pain. It was such a simple solution, and it saved the payer tens of thousands of dollars per year in emergency room visits. You just don't see this happening in our current system.

At the end of the day, addressing social determinants of health to reduce hospital admissions worked. Over a two-year period, readmissions were cut in half, representing more than $3 million in savings for the hospital—more than *three times* what the program cost. Doctors and nurses were not doing this; CHWs making little more than minimum wage were solving these problems.

The success of this program showed that providing care *in* the community by members *of* the community can improve care and reduce costs. It was another great example of value-based care. More than that, we learned it takes more than science to heal people; it takes community, compassion, and *trust*.

A TOUGH SELL

After we proved our community health program could reduce readmissions, we took the show on the road.

Value-based care was in full swing, and payers of all types were looking for ways to reduce costs. One group of payers were *Medicaid Managed Care Organizations* or Medicaid MCOs. Similar to Medicare Advantage, these were private health plans that received money from the government to take better care of Medicaid patients. Our community health program was a perfect match for the problems experienced by Medicaid programs.

At one point, we were able to get a meeting with a Medicaid MCO on the West Coast that was struggling with a high rate of hospitalizations. The executives of the health plan shared data that showed that many of their beneficiaries were using the emergency rooms and hospitals for primary care—and they were often getting readmitted. This was right up our alley. I explained to them the challenges of providing primary care in a population with limited resources and how our program was designed to help manage the most complex patients and keep them out of the hospital.

"How much does it cost?" the CFO asked as we were nearing the end of our presentation.

While my team went back and forth with them about our program's cost, I thought to myself, *How much does it cost you in potentially avoidable hospitalizations every year?* I knew payers like them were getting crushed by people getting constantly admitted—and readmitted—to the hospital for problems we could solve. For sure, our program would save them more than it cost them, just as it did for our other clients. But they seemed disinterested.

At one point, I decided to chime in. "Excuse me, you're the CFO. Your job is to worry about money, right?"

"Right," he said.

"Well, I'm a primary care doctor. My job is to worry about people. The good news is, if you invest in our program and let us take care of your people, you could save a lot of money."

Maybe I was a little direct, but my point was this: if they hired us to help their primary care doctors care for their most complex patients, they could save more money in the long run by reducing potentially avoidable hospitalizations. Unfortunately, my tactic didn't work. We didn't get the job.

Frustrated as we were heading to the airport, I thought to myself—and many times since then—*why doesn't anyone want to pay for primary care anyway?*

THINKING DIFFERENTLY

While value-based care is the right mindset, and policies incentivizing value-based care are the right policies, it has not permeated the landscape. Most doctors are still working in high-volume hospital-based systems, and most primary care is still delivered in an office setting.[55] While there are glimmers of hope—like savings from physician-run ACOs and new Medicare Advantage plans—there has not been a significant change at a national level. Since 2009, national health expenditures have risen from $2.5 trillion to $4.3 trillion in 2021 and are expected to reach nearly $6.2 trillion in 2028.[56] Beyond the money, however, these policies haven't done much to reduce the burden of chronic disease and alleviate human suffering. We need to rely on science for that. But as we discussed, our science is limited.

Reductionism has reduced the human body to trillions of tiny puzzle pieces. And we are pretty good, based on this science, at fixing what goes wrong in the human body—one piece at a time. However, we lack a medical science that pools all of that together from the ground up, from genes to molecules to cells to organs to the whole person sitting in front of us, let alone how that person connects with their families, friends, and community around them.

Just as reductionism is limited, so too is epidemiology. While we have had great successes with large public health programs that solve big problems for lots of people, we lack a science of the individual. Every person is unique and has their own unique set of genes, life experiences, problems, goals, and aspirations. Epidemiology, for all its good in studying populations, does not adequately address the problems of an individual person.

While American medicine has brought us great advances over

the past hundred years, it is insufficient to save us over the next hundred years. If we truly want to solve the problems of our current healthcare system, we need a paradigm shift. We need to look at human beings and our healthcare system for what they really are—*complex systems*.

Part II of this book will take us on a new journey. I will share how I came to understand the nature of complex systems and how it is being applied to human health and disease. We will look at disease as system dysfunction and collapse in response to genetic predisposition and environmental stressors. We will look at medical care in the context of *healing* people, in addition to *fixing* people. Finally, we will look at health as the ability to avoid disease in the first place, rather than simply the absence of disease.

All of this sets the stage for Part III, where we will return to the healthcare system itself. We will consider what a reinvented primary care model could look like; then we will look at how value-based care models could be used to create a truly coordinated healthcare system. After that, we'll take a step back and look at the implications of a coordinated healthcare system for society as a whole. I know it's a bold effort, but what do we have to lose?

My journey into systems thinking and its application to medicine had its roots in an unlikely place—a small hotel cafe in central Florida. It was there that my struggle with a particular theological dilemma collided with my interest in science to produce one of the greatest epiphanies of my life.

PART II

A Paradigm Shift

CHAPTER 5

Systems Thinking

EARLY ONE MORNING, IN THE SPRING OF 2011, I FOUND myself lying in bed in a hotel in central Florida, just staring at the ceiling. I was with my wife, Karen, and daughter, Julia, visiting a local college where Julia had just been accepted as a freshman. I awoke at 4:30 and couldn't get back to sleep. My mind was racing with all kinds of thoughts.

I'm not one to just lie in bed, so I got up and went down to a little cafe. With my notebook in hand, I grabbed a cup of coffee, sat down in a little plastic chair at a small table, and started writing down my thoughts.

What was bothering me?

First up—Easter. Yes, you read that correctly. *Easter!* During my struggles with addiction, I was open to lots of avenues for help, and religion became one of them.

Growing up, my family belonged to an Episcopal church, but

when I married Karen, I converted to her religion—Catholicism. Since they were both Christian religions, I thought I would fit right in. But to be honest, the Catholic church intimidated me. I was not very educated regarding Christian theology; I just had a close relationship with God. But I was fortunate to meet a number of priests and laypeople who made me feel welcome, so I dug in and learned everything I could about Catholicism.

As it happened, that weekend in Florida, I was nearing the end of a thirty-six-week *Ignatian Spiritual Exercise Program*—a set of meditations, contemplations, and prayers written by Saint Ignatius of Loyola, founder of a Catholic Order known as the Jesuits.[57] There were eight very nice people in our group, which was led by an incredible man named John. I loved this group, and they taught me a lot about the ministry of a man called Jesus of Nazareth. But I had one small problem. We were approaching *Easter*—the most important feast of the Christian calendar, marking the resurrection of Jesus three days after his death. That meant I was going to have to share my thoughts on Easter with a group of highly educated Catholics. My insecurities were already starting to come out.

I always had a hard time with Easter. I just couldn't figure out why everyone was so happy. After all, hadn't Jesus just been crucified? Was I the only one sitting there on Easter Sunday still struggling with the events of Good Friday? Why is it even called *Good* Friday? What is good about dying? And what was the Resurrection all about anyway? I mean, I'm a doctor. I had seen people die before. Dead is dead, right? The entire concept of resurrection was difficult for me to comprehend, but frankly, I was too embarrassed to ever talk about it.

But my questions that morning went beyond religion. I had been remarried for five years, my oldest daughter was heading off to college, I was in a solid recovery program, and my new practice was thriving. I thought, *Am I actually on a path to becoming happy?* I wasn't really sure I knew what it meant to be happy. I struggled for most of my life for reasons that were unclear to me. Even when things were going well, I just never seemed to feel…*content.*

All of these thoughts were converging at once. The more I thought about the new direction my life had taken, the more my mind turned away from religion and toward science—specifically, the science of complex systems.

The '80s and '90s saw an increasing number of books written for the general public on complex systems. While I never had any formal training on the subject, I worked through a number of these books in my spare time and in my own way.[58] Some of them were theoretical, and some were practical. Many were full of conjecture, and some were rejected by mainstream science altogether. But they all sought to explore the very nature of our existence and were too enticing to pass up.

It was no surprise that my mind turned to complex systems that morning. I was pondering some big questions, and I needed some big answers. What I didn't know when I sat down in that cafe—but would come to discover years later—was not only would the science of complex systems help me work through big questions in my own life, it would give me insight into how we might tackle our dysfunctional healthcare system in the United States today.

I began to make some connections.

COMPLEX SYSTEMS

Connections—they're everywhere, and they are the essence of complex systems. A system is basically a set of parts connected together to form a distinct entity—a *network*.

Look outside. What do you see? Trees? Flowers? A flock of birds? All of these are systems. Maybe you see cars, buildings, or airplanes. These are systems too—just created by people instead of nature. Have you ever looked up at the clouds in the sky? Or simply felt the wind on your face? The weather is a very complex system. You and every other living thing on the planet Earth are systems, too. Complex biological systems. Make no mistake about it: *systems are everywhere.*

As distinct entities, systems have boundaries. If you are outside a system, you are part of that system's *environment.* Systems interact with their environment constantly, receiving inputs and, in turn, responding to those inputs. I touch a hot stove; I pull my hand back. Pretty simple. But inside a system, there are often a massive number of interacting parts. That's why so many systems are considered *complex.*

Engineers know about systems. They design and build all kinds of systems that perform very specific functions, like rockets, electric grids, and artificial hearts. Ironically, they often limit complexity to build a system that operates in the real world— at least under the conditions it was designed for. For example, consider an airplane. It is designed to fly you safely from one city to another with a reasonable amount of comfort. But what if it encounters bad weather? It might be fine in a small storm, but you certainly wouldn't want to fly in a hurricane. Suffice it to say, it is important to understand the environment in which a system operates.

But to truly appreciate systems, we have to dig a little deeper. What is complexity, and what makes a system *complex*? At its most basic level, simple systems have few parts with few connections, and complex systems have many parts with many connections. In fact, the parts themselves can be systems, creating a *system-of-systems*. While the number of parts might have something to do with the *size* of a system, the number of connections has something to do with the *complexity* of a system. Both are important.

But where does that complexity come from?

While reading these books on complex systems, I became obsessed with something called a random graph. Here's how it goes: imagine you have a thousand buttons on the floor. If I ask you to randomly pick up a button, you pick one button. No surprise there. But if you start randomly connecting those buttons with threads and then randomly pick up a button, you start picking up a bunch of buttons. As you connect more buttons together, a large complex web of buttons forms very quickly. The rapid formation of this new web of buttons is called *emergence*. And like a pop-up thunderstorm on a hot summer day, complex systems can emerge seemingly out of nowhere as individual parts connect together to form new whole entities.

But real systems do not just become complex and stay there

forever. Most complex systems are *dynamic*—they change over time.

Companies are a good example of this. A company often grows from a simple start-up to a very large and complex organization with lots of employees and customers. If economic conditions take a turn for the worse, the company might need to lay off employees, close divisions, and cut off suppliers and vendors. If things get really bad, it might need to simplify things further and declare bankruptcy. Then it might grow back again, restoring connections to suppliers and vendors and reopening whole divisions. It's not uncommon for a company to go from simple to complex, back to simple, and back to complex based on changing economic conditions.

So, if that is system structure, what do we mean by system function?

While the structure of a system might alternate between simple and complex, the function, or behavior, of a system seems to alternate between order and disorder. By order, I mean behavior that is somewhat regular and predictable.

Think of swinging on a swing. You go back and forth, back and forth. The motion is pretty predictable. There is also a certain order to the way our entire world works. The sun rises in the east and sets in the west. The tide comes in and goes out. Birds fly south for the winter and north for the summer. Trees lose their leaves in the fall and regrow them in the spring. Order is nice. Most people like order.

But has your day ever gone to hell in a handbasket? Have you ever thought things were going along just fine, then—*wham!*—

everything falls apart? The behavior of complex systems can be erratic, to say the least. Sometimes we blow it up ourselves.

One of the first books I got on complex systems was *Chaos* by James Gleick, and it changed my whole perspective of our world. We all know chaos when we see it. Just look around at the world today. Do things seem a little chaotic to you? They sure do to me. Sometimes it seems the world is coming apart at the seams. We use the word chaos all the time because it speaks to the craziness in our lives that we can't explain—and that we usually don't want. But in science, the word chaos is generally reserved for a particular type of system dynamic, bizarre but beautiful in its own right.

When we use the word chaos, we usually mean *disorder*—system behavior that is less predictable, haphazard, and sometimes destructive. A hurricane ravages a coastal town. A terrorist bombs a spring concert. Riots fill our city streets. War breaks out in Eastern Europe. Disorder is often uncomfortable. Most people don't like disorder.

At some point, I started thinking about order and disorder in biological systems like my patients—and myself. In biology, we often use the word *homeostasis* to describe the process of maintaining order. It describes how things like body temperature, heart rate, and blood pressure generally stay within certain ranges, like a thermostat regulating the temperature in your house.

We tend to equate order with health, but if that's the case, what about disorder? Does that equate with disease? It certainly seems so. We actually use the word disorder all the time in medicine. When we are not sure exactly what's wrong with a patient, we simply say they have some type of medical disorder.

And how does our environment play into all this? On the one hand, I knew from my epidemiology training that environmental exposures—like smoking, a poor diet, and emotional trauma—put stress on a system and cause disease. On the other hand, not all stress is bad. For example, bone remodels itself under increasing loads, our brain makes new connections based on new experiences, and our muscle cells get bigger with exercise. I saw this firsthand during my days as a physical therapist; I used low amounts of stress to help my patients get stronger and regain their function after an injury.

By now it was about 6:00 a.m. in that small hotel cafe. I sat back in my little plastic chair. Simplicity. Complexity. Order. Disorder. Stress. The whole thing was confusing me and starting to give me a headache. So I stood up, walked around, and got another cup of coffee.

AN EPIPHANY

When I sat back down, I got out some graph paper and started drawing some diagrams to make sense of my thinking. At some point, I decided to draw a graph of structure versus function. This created four quadrants. I asked myself how a system might move around these quadrants in the setting of environmental stressors. It looked something like this:

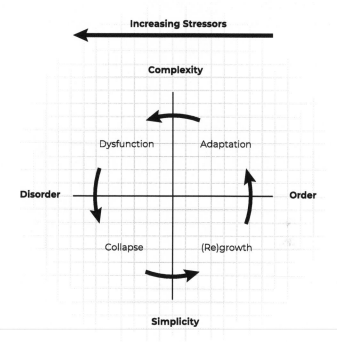

Now that makes sense, I thought. Maybe biological systems cycle through these different quadrants as they navigate environmental stressors. For example, a simple biological system might *grow* in complexity as it increases its number of parts and connections—like the growth of a tree or a child. As a system grows, it might encounter environmental constraints or stressors. In response, the system might *adapt* to the changing conditions, all the while increasing its complexity by increasing and rearranging its connections. But if the stressors continued, the behavior might become *dysfunctional*, and the system could start to fall apart. If the stressors continued further, the system might get pushed past some tipping point and *collapse*

altogether, back into a more simple structure. With fewer connections and less stress, the system could reorganize itself and *regrow*—starting the cycle all over again.

Growth, adaptation, dysfunction, collapse, and regrowth. It seemed obvious enough. I sat there and looked at my graph. True, it was pure conjecture, vastly oversimplified, and maybe completely wrong, but there was something pleasing and familiar about it. Then it hit me: *This is what happened to me. This is a model of my life!*

I grew up in a small town northeast of Philadelphia. I adapted to the physical, mental, and social challenges I faced to reach peak health just before medical school. Then, ten years of stress—massive stress from multiple sources—caused my body to break down on many levels. Then one prescription drug did me in. I got caught in a self-inflicted feedback loop, and I collapsed like a house of cards.

But the story didn't end there. I pressed on. I *simplified* my life and healed from my physical and emotional injuries. Once healed, I changed course and *rebuilt* my life—physically, mentally, and socially. Now here I was, in a hotel in Central Florida with my wife and daughter, getting ready to share what would be one of many beautiful memories in my *new life*. Finally, everything seemed to make sense.

Then, something very strange happened. I started thinking about all my friends in recovery and how we all have our own *rock bottom*—the point at which we can't take it anymore and from which, if we survive, we change course and rebuild our lives. But I knew everyone's rock bottom was different. Some people have "lower" bottoms than others. I knew for a fact there were others who had it much worse than me. I wondered, *How low does the bottom of this graph go anyway? How low could someone get and still be able to turn it around?*

I started drawing deeper U-shaped arrows and extending the vertical line of my graph lower and lower, all the while thinking of my friends in recovery who experienced much worse trauma than me. Physical, sexual, and emotional abuse. Homelessness. Discrimination. Starvation. Incarceration. Yet they would all go on to rebuild their lives, too.

Then, as I extended the vertical line down further, out of nowhere, my graph slowly turned into a cross. A big, beautiful, radiant cross. Suddenly, it hit me like a bolt of lightning—suffering, death, and *resurrection*!

I felt a pit in my stomach. *Holy shit,* I thought. *So that's what the Resurrection is all about.* I had been so focused on the details of Good Friday, I completely missed the meaning of Easter Sunday! And that is this: *death is not only the end of something old, it can be the beginning of something new.*

I just sat there and shook my head. After all these years, I could finally appreciate the beauty and joy of Easter Sunday. Ironically, it took science to teach it to me. To this day, I see resurrections everywhere, all the time. They are beautiful and joyous, indeed.

It turns out, I wasn't the only one thinking about complex systems and how they could be applied to biological systems. Unbeknownst to me, a new field called systems biology was in full swing at the time. This new science would look at biological systems in a whole new way—from the bottom up, rather than the top down. It would investigate how cells function as a *system,* and it would use new technology and computer modeling to do so.

SYSTEMS BIOLOGY: A NEW SCIENCE

There's a joke that if you ask three people to define systems biology, you'll get seven different answers. But let's give it a shot. At its most basic level, systems biology is the attempt to bring different fields together to truly understand how a biological system works. You can't just look at the properties of one small piece of a system. You need to understand that piece in context; you need to understand how the pieces interact with each other and with their local environment.[59]

To achieve a deeper understanding of how biological systems function, systems biology merges three different fields together: mathematics, computer science, and biology. By combining these fields, scientists hope to move beyond reductionism to understand how organisms work as a system. If we only look at a cell by itself, we're missing the bigger picture—that the cell is part of an organ, which is part of an organism, which interacts with the environment around it.

How does systems biology assemble those parts within a system? How does it study a system's interaction with its environment? That's where computer science and mathematics come in. By simulating how system properties change over time, computational models are a way that we can understand and maybe even predict the behavior of a complex system.

At first, researchers may not have any actual data to work with, so they will often start by putting sample data into a mathematical model—a process called *estimation*. Then they can use the results of the model to design a real experiment and generate real data. The real data can be fed back into the model and the model can be adjusted, again and again. This technique is called *iteration*, and as in life itself, it is a very powerful method to improve predictions about how a system might respond to a change in environmental conditions over time.

What kind of data do system biologists model? New technologies allow scientists to measure massive numbers of molecules very quickly. When molecules from certain systems are grouped together and studied, they are given the suffix *-omics*. For example, studying a group of genes is called genomics, studying a group of proteins is called proteomics, and so on. Systems biology models how biological elements interact with each other over time.

But systems biology also considers how environmental exposures affect system structure and function. As a group, these exposures are called, not surprisingly, *exposomics*. These include environmental toxins for sure, but they could include any type of exposure from physical and biological to psychological and social. Environmental exposures can put stress on biological systems—as such they can also be called *environmental stressors*. I'll have a lot more to say about environmental stressors in the next chapter, but suffice it to say, they are important.

Systems biology, with all its technology and computational power, holds great promise. But how does systems biology translate into the care of patients? How do we go from computational models to clinical medicine? While there are many fields that take a systems approach to healthcare, I will use the term *systems medicine* to tie them all together.

SYSTEMS MEDICINE

The fact that a group of genes can interact with a group of molecules to form a living cell is mind-boggling enough. But how do those cells interact and self-organize to form organs like your heart, lungs, and kidneys? Furthermore, how do those organs interact and self-organize to form you as a human being? You are indeed a *system-of-systems*. And like that pop-up thunderstorm on a hot summer day, *you* as a human being actually emerge from the underlying networks of genes, molecules, cells, and organs inside you.

Systems medicine has many definitions, but at its core, it seeks to understand human health and disease as emergent properties of a network of interacting molecules within you. As such, it is related to a field called network medicine.[60] It's not based on a science of reductionism alone. It is also based on a science of *holism*—a science that seeks to understand you as a *whole person*.[61] It can do this by looking at data from multiple sources at multiple levels, including the *-omics* technologies discussed earlier and physiological data from new wearable devices. In fact, computational modeling of physiological data is often called systems physiology.[62] But beyond -omics and physiological data, systems medicine can also include data from human performance, self-perception, and environmental exposures. All of these data sources can be used to understand you as a complex biological system and how you interact with the environment around you.[63]

Collecting and modeling all this information is no easy task, and it's fair to say that this field is still in its infancy, even though the concept has been around for over twenty years. One early version of systems medicine—championed by Dr. Leroy Hood—is referred to as "P4 Medicine," since it is predictive, preventive, personalized, and participatory in its mission.[64] It's *predictive* in that computational power enables physicians to predict the probability of disease based on large amounts of data from individual patients. It's *preventive* because it can identify contributing factors to disease and potential interventions to mitigate a disease process. It is *personalized* because medical recommendations can be made specific to an individual patient. Finally, it is *participatory* because it invites the patient to participate in their care. While the concepts of systems medicine continue to evolve, these core principles remain relevant to its overall mission.

Systems medicine is related to a field called *precision medicine*, sometimes referred to as "personalized medicine." It typically uses personalized data—particularly genomic data—to tailor medical treatments to individual patients.[65] Once the human genome could be sequenced in the early 2000s, genomics began to be used to inform drug dosing decisions based on a patient's genes—a field called *pharmacogenomics*. The precision medicine movement got a boost in 2015 when President Barack Obama signed the "Precision Medicine Initiative," which provided funding through the NIH to study applications of precision medicine for various diseases. Advances in precision medicine have already led to new discoveries and several treatments that are tailored to a person's genetic makeup, or the genetic profile of an individual's cancer.[66] Precision medicine will play a big role in a reinvented primary care model. We'll talk about that in more detail in Chapter 9.

But systems medicine goes beyond pharmacogenomics and the individualized treatment of disease to consider the effects of the broader environment on whole system function—from the air we breathe to the food we eat to the way we live our lives.[67] With such an approach to patient care, systems medicine overlaps with the clinical fields of osteopathic medicine, integrative medicine, lifestyle medicine, functional medicine, and even the entire health and fitness industry. These groups are less concerned about the use of pharmacologic interventions to restore health and more interested in *lifestyle interventions*—nutrition, exercise, sleep, and the nature of relationships with other people. The challenge with these fields, however, is that they are extremely diverse, less regulated, and do not always meet the rigorous standards of conventional medicine research.

Of course, it's not that conventional medicine ignores lifestyle interventions. The American Heart Association, in particular, provides extensive evidence-based recommendations on how to reduce your risk of cardiovascular disease using lifestyle interventions.[68] Likewise, the CDC offers lifestyle programs to reduce the risk of diabetes.[69]

Suffice it to say all these fields speak to the same underlying philosophy: *the way we live our life has a direct impact on our health and risk of disease.* I'll have a lot more to say about how we can use lifestyle interventions to improve our health in Chapter 8.

A NEW FRAMEWORK

The term "systems medicine" basically refers to a construct for looking at patients as complex systems living in a complex environment. It's a different way to think about health and human disease, and I believe it could help us improve patient care.

But could the principles of systems medicine also improve the healthcare system itself? Could it help create a coordinated and effective healthcare system for everyone? It turns out, systems-based models have already been proposed for healthcare transformation.[70] And the American Medical Association is embracing "health systems science" as the future of medicine and medical education.[71] By taking a systems approach to solving our complex healthcare problem, maybe there is hope for turning things around after all.

I am optimistic that systems medicine can help get us out of the healthcare conundrum we discussed in Part I of this book. But some big questions still remain. *How would systems medicine be integrated into a multitrillion dollar sickcare system? Could it possibly serve as a framework for value-based care and reduce the burden of disease in this country?* Maybe it can.

But before we can tackle those big questions, we need to get back to the basics. *What do we even mean by the word disease, anyway?*

That would be a question I wrestled with after meeting a young woman named Stephanie.

CHAPTER 6

Redefining Disease

STEPHANIE WAS A TWENTY-ONE-YEAR-OLD WOMAN I MET during my fellowship at Hopkins. She was the daughter of a friend of mine, and my friend asked if I would be her primary care doctor. I told her of course I would; I was building my sports medicine practice and was happy to bring on new patients. But Stephanie was not a typical referral to my practice at the time. She had a unique situation—she had a genetic disease called Turner Syndrome.

Turner Syndrome occurs when one of the two X chromosomes in a female is partially or completely absent.[72] Since the X chromosome contains many genes needed for normal growth and development, patients with Turner Syndrome often develop differently. This became apparent with Stephanie around the age of eight when she was not growing at the rate of other girls her age. Turner Syndrome, like many genetic conditions, comes with a laundry list of potential abnormalities—short stature, infertility, heart defects, kidney defects, bone problems, eye problems, hearing issues. When someone is diagnosed with Turner Syndrome, it can be devastating.

I had never seen a case of Turner Syndrome before, and I am not a geneticist. So I did what any intellectually insecure physician would do: I read everything I could about Turner Syndrome before I saw Stephanie. *This is going to be complicated,* I thought to myself. *So many things could be wrong here.*

While Stephanie sat in the waiting room with her friend, I took a deep breath and walked out to get her. What I found were two young women talking and laughing with each other. Honestly, I'm not exactly sure what I was expecting. I made some small talk, then brought Stephanie back to my office. The whole time, I was thinking, *She looks like a normal young woman to me.*

Stephanie and I talked for a while about her family and her life. Her story was remarkable for what wasn't there—no illnesses, no injuries, no medical problems except some expected endocrine issues, which were perfectly treated. The only issue, and it was significant, was that she was infertile.

On examination, Stephanie seemed athletic, despite the fact that she did not exercise. And her blood work was exquisite—I had actually never seen anything quite like it. At the end of the visit, I had to make sense of this whole experience. The person I had gotten to know over those couple of hours was not who I was expecting.

Trying to recover from my initial bias, yet wanting to be honest about her situation, I said to her, "Stephanie, you are an incredibly healthy young woman. I don't want to minimize the issue of not having kids, because that has to be difficult. But one way or another, you are going to make a great mom." Then I went on, "Sure, you have this one little genetic issue over here. But you have over twenty thousand perfectly normal genes that make you who you are—an incredibly healthy and athletic young woman."

Stephanie looked at me and said, "I'm not an athlete. My sisters are the athletes."

I said, "But you can be an athlete. You can be anything you want to be. As I look at your blood work, you are not just genetically normal, you are genetically *gifted!* Your ability to metabolize energy and build muscle is incredible. You just have to challenge your body to do it!"

It didn't occur to me at the time, but Stephanie had never thought of herself as athletic. She always lived in the shadows of her two older sisters, who were, in fact, accomplished athletes. She certainly never thought of herself as genetically gifted; all her life, she felt defined by her genetic condition.

Later that day, her mom called to thank me. Apparently, for the first time ever, Stephanie felt good about her health. Honestly, I felt embarrassed that I almost missed the opportunity to have a positive impact on Stephanie because I was so worried about the details of her genetic condition.

The whole situation made me rethink the concept of disease and reminded me of a quote from Sir William Osler: "It is much more important to know what sort of a patient has a disease than what sort of a disease a patient has."[73] In this case, the "disease" of Turner Syndrome had nothing over a young woman named Stephanie.

WHAT IS A DISEASE?

We talked a lot about chronic diseases in Chapter 2, such as hypertension, obesity, diabetes, mental illness, and heart disease. Chronic disease, it seems, is everywhere. But what exactly is chronic disease? What do we even mean by the word *disease*?

Unfortunately, nowadays diseases seem to have become mere labels based on population data and established cut-off points. Hemoglobin A1C 6.5 percent? Congratulations, you have diabetes! Blood pressure 130 over 80? Congratulations, you have hypertension! By categorizing diseases like this, we have oversimplified them.

Chronic diseases are much more complicated. They are dynamic processes that evolve over time. They often involve a deviation from normal physiological function, or a loss of homeostasis. As such, many diseases can be thought of as disordered function, or dysfunction, of a complex biological system.

But chronic diseases do not arise out of nowhere. We know from over a century of epidemiology that diseases are often caused by environmental exposures that put stress on the human body—exposures such as air pollution, chemical toxins, infections, emotional trauma, and poor diet. In fact, sometimes a disease might not even be a disease at all; it might simply be the body's attempt to adapt to a chronic environmental stressor.[74]

Type 2 diabetes is a good example. If I eat more sugar than my body can handle—say because I am not very active—that sugar can easily be converted to fat. That fat can, in turn, block the ability of sugar to get into my muscle cells.[75] As a result, my blood sugar rises. It's almost as if my muscle cells are trying to protect themselves from all the sugar I'm eating! Unless I reduce my sugar intake and become more active, my body will accumulate more fat and my blood sugar will rise further. In other words, my diabetes gets worse. Left unchecked, this process can cause all kinds of other problems, like kidney disease, heart disease, nerve damage, or loss of vision.

The course a disease takes over time is often called its *trajectory*. Sometimes diseases progress quickly; sometimes they progress slowly. That begs the question: *why does the same disease behave differently in different people?*

Systems medicine suggests that diseases emerge from the bottom up—from genes to molecules to cells to organs to whole people living in an environment full of various stressors. But disease is not just about environmental stressors; it's about the wrong stressors in the wrong person. What do I mean by that? I mean that a person's genes are at play here.

Sometimes the process of copying genes from parent to child goes wrong and a gene develops a *mutation*—an abnormality in gene structure. This is what happened to my patient Stephanie. Of course, sometimes a genetic mutation combined with an environmental stressor might lead to a disease and sometimes it might not. In fact, sometimes, a mutation might even protect us from a disease.[76] Our genes are constantly interacting with our environment and affecting our health. In other words, it's not nature or nurture—its nature *and* nurture.

I liken the gene-environment interaction to playing a game of poker. You can be dealt a bad hand, but if you play it really well and have a little luck, you can win big. Conversely, you could be dealt an incredible hand—even four aces! But if you play it poorly, you can lose your shirt.

Life is like playing poker with over twenty thousand cards, and no two hands are ever the same. Unless you have an identical twin, your set of genes is unlike anyone else who has ever existed. This is thanks to something called genetic variation.

GENETIC VARIANTS

We've all heard the phrase "everybody is unique," right? That's thanks to genetic *variants*. Variants are not mutations, per se. They are normal genes that have a slightly different structure from person to person. Given the size of the human genome, 3.2 billion base pairs total, the number of combinations of variants is nearly infinite.[77]

So where did these variants come from? Why isn't everyone exactly the same? Genetic variants came about because they offered a survival advantage in some environment at some point in human history—or at least, they were not a disadvantage.[78]

There are a lot of reasons why a genetic variant might be advantageous to someone in a particular environment. For example, the variant that causes sickle cell anemia also reduces the risk of dying from malaria. That was great if you lived in a malaria-infested region of Africa seven thousand years ago.[79] But it doesn't help much in current day North America, where malaria is not a problem.

Lactose intolerance is another example. That one came from populations that went rapidly from hunting and gathering to farming. Farming populations retained the ability to process lactose, whereas hunter-gatherers did not.[80] So if you are a descendant of hunter-gatherers instead of farmers, you might have a problem drinking milk.

We all have some combination of genetic variants that allows us to function really well in certain environments but not so well in others. The problem is, apart from these very obvious examples, we generally don't know what those environments are. We're all essentially flying blind. If we are genetically wired for a certain set of environmental conditions but we are thrown into a different environment, chances are we are going to have a problem.

So are we completely at the mercy of our genes? Well, yes and no. Of course, we can't change our genetic makeup (although there is a very interesting technology called CRISPR that could change all that).[81] *But we can make changes to the way we live our lives in order to better match what our genes are looking for.*

Let's take a look at how environmental stressors can affect the human body so that we can better understand *why* it's so critical to reduce them.

STRESSORS AND TIPPING POINTS

In Chapter 2, I told a story about a patient of mine named Faith. She had been developing symptoms of an autoimmune disease that defied a diagnosis for years. When she came to me, I sent her to see a doctor friend of mine, a specialist. He told her that he thought her symptoms were due to stress. Faith was upset with that idea, and rightly so. To her, it was the old *it's all in your head* argument.

That specialist certainly could have phrased it differently, but the truth is, he was kind of right. Faith was suffering from the *effects* of stress—years and years of multiple environmental stressors that eventually pushed her past a tipping point into an actual disease state. In her case, it was an autoimmune disease. But it could have been a heart attack, cancer, or even suicide.

Our modern American healthcare system is geared to look for one solution to one problem at a time. A broken bone. Appendicitis. Pneumonia. We can fix those problems. But chronic diseases are not that easy; chronic diseases are often complex conditions caused by a multitude of contributing factors. These factors can add up and put cumulative stress on the system. Yes, Faith had a very real autoimmune disease that needed to be treated, but to truly help her and the millions of people like her, we need to address not just the problem at hand, but also the multitude of factors causing physiological dysfunction and eventually pushing a system past a tipping point.

Tipping points, or critical thresholds, have been the subject of a number of books related to complex systems.[82] They describe a very sudden and dramatic shift in system behavior under increasing amounts of stress. Think about an avalanche. You're looking at a mountain top, at all the snow that has accumulated as stored energy. It doesn't really look like much is going on. It's actually quite beautiful—until one day, a little more snow falls high up on the mountain. Next thing you know, half of the mountain comes crashing down with enormous energy. And that avalanche is not stopping until it has reached its lowest local energy state. In the process, a lot of damage might get done.

Conceptually, the same thing can happen in humans. Think of a heart attack. That's kind of like an avalanche inside an artery around your heart caused by twenty years of accumulated energy in the form of a "lipid plaque."

A lipid plaque is a small but complex molecular structure formed in response to environmental stressors in a genetically susceptible person. If the stressors accumulate, the plaque can become unstable and cause a heart attack. What triggered the heart attack? Sometimes it's obvious like shoveling snow or fighting with a friend. But that's just the end game. The triggering event was really just the final straw in a lifetime of cumulative stressors: work, smoking, poor diet, sedentary lifestyle, the list goes on.

It turns out there are some pretty simple mathematical models that describe the behavior of a system as it approaches a tipping point.[83] And, as we'll see later on, I believe we can harness the power of these models to detect and treat disease early in the process—long before it causes significant damage.

This points to one of the central roles of primary care. Part of my job as a doctor is to help you understand your genetic makeup, then help you determine what environmental exposures are uniquely bad for you—what exposures you really need to stay away from—and what environmental exposures might be good for you—those that can actually improve your health. Generally speaking, there is no rulebook when it comes to what is good and bad for you, since everyone has a unique genetic background. What's good for me might be bad for you and vice-versa.

We typically use the word stress in the singular sense. But in reality, stress can come in a variety of different forms. Let's take a closer look at some different types of environmental stressors humans face to better understand how they affect us—and how they could push us past a tipping point.

PHYSICAL STRESSORS

Living on planet Earth can be stressful, even dangerous. We are bombarded with physical stressors on a daily basis, most of which we take for granted.

Let's start with gravity. We don't think about gravity that much, but it can cause all kinds of problems. Over 32 million people suffer from arthritis in this country.[84] Osteoarthritis is caused by the thinning of cartilage due to the compressive effects of gravity on joints, such as the knee and hip and spine. Poor posture and body mechanics only make the situation worse. Have you ever had swelling in your feet? That's gravity keeping fluid from returning to your heart. We also have a $27 billion plastic surgery industry, much of which exists to fix the effects of gravity on our skin.[85] The problem with gravity is that you can't get away from it—unless, of course, you go into outer space, but as we'll see, that causes a whole other set of problems.

Gravity isn't the only physical stressor on our planet. We are also bombarded with electromagnetic radiation on a daily basis. Anyone who has had a sunburn, or a skin cancer that results from it, knows about the effects of radiation.

How about light itself? For four billion years, life has evolved on this planet in alternating cycles of day and night. As humans, we have developed *circadian rhythms*—our natural response to the cycle of light and dark.[86] But once the light bulb was invented, we created one of the greatest stressors that human beings have ever known. At midnight, we can find ourselves in a brightly lit room or staring at a bright computer screen. That's not normal. Our bodies want to sleep, but we're awake.

Another physical stressor is the weather itself. For example, earlier today I went *rucking*—basically hiking with a heavy backpack. It was extremely hot outside, so my body naturally started to sweat to cool itself off. After a while I was sweating profusely and started getting thirsty, so I stopped to rest in the shade and drink some water. If I didn't take a break I could eventually have suffered a *heat stroke*—a potentially lethal condition from being overheated, like a car with a broken radiator.

Heat stroke is a major concern in athletes training or competing in the heat of summer. On average, 658 people die every year in the US from heat-related illness.[87] Cold temperatures can be even more dangerous. Without proper clothing in severely cold weather, the body cannot maintain normal body temperature. In fact, about 1,300 people die annually from hypothermia.[88]

But it's more than just temperature that causes us stress. There are natural disasters like thunderstorms, tornadoes, hurricanes, and floods. Think of the stress those events have on the families and communities impacted by them.

Sometimes we cause our own physical stress as we try to improve our health. Recently a patient of mine was training for a marathon and developed a *stress fracture*—small fractures of a bone, often due to repeated impact with the ground. She was so determined to run this marathon, she gave it only a week of rest before she went back to running.

When this patient saw me, she said, "My foot still hurts."

I said, "Well, are you resting it?"

"No," she replied, "but I backed off on my runs. I'm going slower."

"You're running on a stress fracture?" I asked. "You can't do that. You have to allow it time to heal."

I guess this patient didn't understand that she couldn't just push her way through it. Or maybe she didn't want to understand. Some of us are addicted to exercise to the point that we actually cause ourselves harm.

The good news is that we can adapt to many of these physical stressors, as long as they are introduced gradually. Adaptation to stress is the key to good health and, frankly, our survival as a species. We'll discuss more about how we can harness the power of adaptation in Chapter 8.

CHEMICAL TOXINS

Earlier, we talked about possibly the greatest chemical toxin to humans in modern society: sugar. While sugar can be a source of energy for the human body, in high doses and with the wrong genes, it can be toxic, causing type 2 diabetes. Smoking is another voluntary source of chemical toxins. When burned, a cigarette creates more than seven thousand chemicals, sixty-nine of which are known to cause cancer.[89] But it's not just sugar and cigarettes that can do us in. Every day, our bodies are bombarded by all kinds of chemical toxins.

Toxins are everywhere—in the air that we breathe, the water we drink, and the food we eat—and they can have a negative impact on our health. Pesticides and herbicides are toxins, along with other man-made chemicals and heavy metals that find their way into our air, soil, and water. And then there are plastics. Tiny plastic particles called *microplastics* are everywhere—from the bottom of our deepest oceans to the top of Mount Everest—and we are only just beginning to understand their negative impact on human health.[90]

Sometimes, the body makes its own toxins as a product of normal metabolism. A good example of this is a *free radical*—a highly unstable molecule that can damage organs in the body such as heart, lungs, and kidneys. While there are health benefits to free radicals, such as in fighting infections, excess free radicals can have negative effects.[91] To avoid these negative effects, we have to neutralize them with antioxidants obtained from a healthy diet.

Finally, we have our beloved medications. We don't think of medications as toxins, but as we saw in Chapter 2, they can be harmful or even deadly. On the other hand they can be life-saving. It is for this reason that medical providers, such as physicians, nurse practitioners, and physician assistants, require training in *pharmacology*—a field that teaches us how to prescribe medications appropriately. Having a license to prescribe medications is an incredible privilege. One that I don't take lightly.

Thankfully for us, the human body has an amazing capacity to metabolize and eliminate toxins, including the medications we prescribe to our patients. In fact, much of my pharmacology course in medical school was dedicated to how the liver and kidneys metabolize and eliminate toxins. The liver is one of the most spectacular organs in the human body. Not only does it manufacture many important molecules, it can make many toxins water-soluble so that they can get filtered out by our kidneys. As long as we keep our exposure to toxins low and incorporate the right nutrients into our diet, our bodies can handle most toxins just fine.

A WORLD OF BUGS

There's been an incredible war going on for millions of years between the human immune system and the biological world around us—and it's still raging in each and every one of us to this day. Usually we don't know it's even happening. It's only when something like COVID-19 comes along that the war comes to the forefront of everyone's brain.

In reality, every second of every day, we live amongst trillions of viruses, bacteria, worms, and other parasites. Trust me, you don't want to know what's on your skin, let alone in your gut!

Our bodies coexist with what is called a *microbiome*—a massive ecosystem of microorganisms that we carry along with us all the time.

The microbiome is getting a lot of attention these days, for good reason—it's massive. There are an estimated one hundred times more bacterial and viral genes available for metabolism in the human gut than there are genes in the human genome.[92] Epidemiology and systems biology suggest that our microbiome has important roles in training our immune system, digesting our food, regulating hormones, signaling neurons, metabolizing drugs, eliminating toxins, and producing numerous compounds that influence our health. Furthermore, it appears that changes in the gut microbiome are associated with diseases such as obesity, diabetes, liver disease, and cardiometabolic disease.[93] We are learning more and more about the microbiome every day, but it's fair to say there is much more that we *don't know* about this ecosystem than we *do know* at this point.

As a general rule, people with a well-regulated immune system and healthy microbiome can fend off most infections. In fact, many infections, such as sinus infections, urinary tract infections, skin infections, and gut infections, probably do not need to be treated with antibiotics at all. Antibiotics are already overprescribed in this country.[94]

Our immune system has an incredible capacity to neutralize infectious agents, just like chemical toxins. With notable exceptions (such as the COVID-19 virus), it's fair to say we have a pretty good relationship with the biological world around us.

COGNITIVE OVERLOAD

You're overcommitted at work and you are asked to take on another project. You don't want to disappoint your colleagues, so you agree. You push yourself harder because you have to be done by five to make dinner by six and get to your child's recital by eight.

Or maybe it's the opposite problem. You spent thousands of dollars and four years of your life to get a college degree. Now you are spending all day looking for a job—filling out applications and going to interviews—but no one is hiring. By the time you go to bed you're exhausted but can't fall asleep. You have a pit in your stomach and your heart is pounding. All you can think is, *How am I going to get through all this?*

When we talk about stress, we are usually talking about *psychological stress*—stress that results from navigating the demands of our modern life. Left unchecked, psychological stress can lead to anxiety and even clinical depression.[95]

When we are faced with too many tasks at one time, our sympathetic nervous system gets activated and we feel overwhelmed by a sense of fear and anxiety. Then the smallest thing can set us off. We instinctively have a *fight, flight, or freeze response*—we either act aggressively, run away, or stand there like a deer in a headlight. This response isn't always a bad thing. In fact, thousands of years ago, acute stress probably helped us survive as a species.[96] The real problem is *chronic stress*—constant pressure that consumes us on a day-to-day basis.

Chronic psychological stress is corrosive. It can lead to the constant production of stress hormones, such as cortisol. While cortisol is great in an emergency, it's not good in high levels for long periods of time. It can cause all kinds of problems, including anxiety, depression, digestive problems, headaches, muscle pain, high blood pressure, insomnia, weight gain, and poor memory.[97]

Unfortunately chronic stress is everywhere. Think about all that information you are getting from television or social media. Everywhere you turn there is a problem or conflict. Is there anything good going on in the world? No matter how you look at it, chronic psychological stress is not good for the human body. Somehow, we have to figure out a way to reduce this pervasive and often unnecessary stressor.

EMOTIONAL TRAUMA

As a primary care doctor, I develop close relationships with my patients. This in turn allows patients to feel comfortable opening up to me. As a result, I have heard a lot of stories and worked with many patients who have experienced deep emotional trauma. Children who have committed suicide. Loved ones who have overdosed on drugs or alcohol. Survivors of physical, sexual, and emotional abuse. These kinds of trauma are hard to compare with the psychological stress of making too many appointments. They are, in my opinion, qualitatively different.

Emotional trauma, I have found, often pushes people past a tipping point. It can act like a tidal wave that capsizes a boat. I don't have objective evidence that emotional trauma causes acute illness, but I don't have to—I've seen it firsthand. Twice in my career, I have seen a husband die and a week later the wife dies unexpectedly—one after sixty years of marriage.

In the most recent situation, the wife had a massive stroke a week after her husband died from cancer. Was that a coincidence? Not in my book. I spoke with her every day after her husband died. I tried to tell her everything would be okay. But she was devastated. Her husband was her soulmate. Perhaps people really can die of a broken heart.

Somehow we have to move on after a tragedy, which means we have to learn to live and cope with the pain that results. Yet this isn't always as easy as it sounds. Many people suffer from *Post-Traumatic Stress Disorder (PTSD)*—a condition that may occur in people who have experienced or witnessed a traumatic event. We often see this with our Veteran community, many of whom have experienced significant trauma during times of war. Others suffer from a *moral injury*—engaging in or witnessing behaviors that go against an individual's core values or moral beliefs.[98] These experiences embed deep memories, which can suddenly resurface in a grocery store or the middle of the night years down the road.

But there is treatment. It's usually not a litany of drugs that can sometimes cause more problems but real therapy by qualified and compassionate therapists—often Veterans themselves who have been through similar situations.[99]

RESOURCE SCARCITY

In Chapter 4, I told you about a community health program we created to reduce readmissions to a local community hospital. We were successful by helping people get the community resources they needed to better manage their health problems.

So why do people with fewer resources typically have poorer

health? In part, because we need resources to help us manage other environmental stressors. Without access to adequate housing, nutritious food, clean water, employment opportunities, and reliable transportation, all other stressors will be compounded, leading to potential health consequences. Add to that the stress of discrimination and marginalization, and the situation only gets worse.

Let's take a quick look at resource scarcity and how it can amplify other stressors—starting with housing. An increasing body of evidence has associated poor housing quality with morbidity from infectious diseases, chronic illnesses, injuries, poor nutrition, and mental health disorders.[100] For example, without air conditioning or heat, people can suffer from the physical stressors of heat-related illnesses or hypothermia. Furthermore, housing for economically disadvantaged people might be sited near hazardous industrial plants, increasing people's exposure to chemical toxins and air pollution. Finally, many families in public housing are packed into tighter living spaces, which could allow pathogens to proliferate more easily, leading to more infections. Regardless of the details, it is fair to say adequate and safe housing is important for good health.

Lack of transportation is another issue. In fact, it was one of the biggest issues in our community health program. What happened when one of our patients didn't have a car or access to public transportation? They struggled to maintain a job to support an income. They had difficulty visiting friends and became socially isolated. Or they were unable to get to a doctor when they needed care. Many of us take for granted our ability to move around our communities, but when our transportation is restricted, we are unable to utilize other community resources important to maintaining our health.

Even this is just the tip of the iceberg. What about the lack of access to nutritious food? Noise pollution from traffic leading to sleepless nights? High crime rates causing people to live in fear for their lives?

Some people live with stressors that feed back on each other, causing a cycle of hospitalizations. For example, mold in the walls sends a child to the hospital because they're having an asthma attack. Hospital bills add up, and the family can't afford air conditioning, making the mold problem worse and causing more asthma attacks. Back to the hospital they go.[101]

Every day, people are living in environments where they don't have the proper resources to live a healthy life or protect themselves from other environmental stressors. They can easily get caught up in a web of despair based on socioeconomic stressors alone, which in turn open the door to all other stressors—compounding one on top of the other. If we really want to reduce the burden of chronic disease in this country and the high costs that come with it, we are going to have to ensure people have access to the resources they need to improve their health.

WHAT STRESSES YOU OUT?

Everyone has a few of these stressors, if not more. What are yours? What stressors are you accumulating that will lead you to physical or psychological dis-ease down the road?

I've argued that chronic disease is caused by excessive environmental stressors in genetically susceptible people. But identifying all the genetic and environmental factors that contribute to the development of disease is extremely difficult. There is just no way you can figure all this out on your own, and unfortunately our current hospital-based healthcare system isn't designed to help you.

As we'll see in the next chapter, our healthcare system is pretty good at fixing people with acute injuries and illnesses, but not so good at helping people heal from chronic diseases that cause so much suffering.

No one taught me this lesson more than a patient of mine named Joe.

CHAPTER 7

Fixing *and* Healing

JOE WAS A FIFTY-YEAR-OLD MAN WHO WAS REFERRED TO me by mutual friends after he had difficulty recovering from a heart attack. Prior to his appointment, I had some pretty detailed medical records to review—including records from the paramedics, emergency department, local hospital, and other physicians. Let me tell you his story as I learned it from the medical records.

Joe worked in finance and was a husband and father of two girls. He was also an avid exerciser, running four to five miles a day, six days a week without any trouble. He had little in the way of medical history except for some high cholesterol, which ran in his family. By all accounts, Joe seemed *healthy*.

One day after returning home from a five-mile run, Joe felt a strange pressure in his chest. He didn't pay too much attention to it, attributing it to the food he ate for lunch before his run. Then, out of nowhere, his breathing became labored and he started to feel lightheaded. He broke out in a sweat and became nauseous. His wife, who was home at the time, immediately called 911.

When the paramedics arrived, they found Joe lying on the floor sweating profusely and breathing rapidly. His oxygen level was low at 85 percent. His blood pressure was extremely low at 85/40. His pulse was rapid and irregular. Then he lost consciousness.

The paramedics immediately applied a defibrillator and gave him an electric shock. Then another. Joe came to. His blood pressure improved, but he still had severe chest pain and shortness of breath. They immediately did an EKG, which showed *ST elevation*—a sign of a massive heart attack. They gave him oxygen, aspirin, and nitroglycerine and immediately transported him to a nearby hospital with an advanced cardiovascular center.

At the hospital, Joe received state-of-the-art medical care, including emergent *cardiac catheterization*—a procedure where they place a catheter into the coronary arteries and look for a blocked artery. Joe did, in fact, have a complete blockage of his Left Anterior Descending (LAD) artery—otherwise known as the "widow-maker" because patients so often die from such a blockage. The blockage was due to a blood clot, caused by cholesterol plaque that had ruptured in his artery. Joe's "avalanche" came crashing down in a matter of minutes. Fortunately, the cardiologist was able to open the blocked artery and place a stent. Blood flow was restored in less than an hour. Joe's blocked artery was fixed.

Joe was admitted to the Coronary Care Unit or CCU, where

his heart could be closely monitored. The fluid in his lungs, his high blood pressure, and his high cholesterol were all controlled with medications. Joe made a remarkable recovery. He was eventually transferred to a step-down unit and discharged home a few days later. This was American medicine at its best.

With his host of new medications and some cardiac rehab, Joe got back to his normal life pretty quickly—a life of fast-paced business deals, poor sleep, and exercising six days a week to cope with all the stress at work. But something wasn't quite right.

First, Joe never got his energy back after he got home from the hospital. Then, he developed occasional lightheadedness and the strange feeling of "brain fog." He saw his primary care doctor, who sent him to a series of specialists—an endocrinologist prescribed testosterone, a gastroenterologist prescribed an antacid medicine, and a psychiatrist prescribed an antidepressant. But nothing worked.

It wasn't long afterward that Joe came to see me. After I reviewed his records, and before I even saw him, one thing was immediately clear to me—nothing was going to fix Joe. Joe needed to *heal*.

Hospitals are good at fixing people; they are just not so good at *healing* people. As we'll see, healing is a process best guided by primary care providers who have relationships with their patients. But the physician-patient relationship has been damaged by a reimbursement system that forces doctors to see a large number of patients, which prevents time to establish a relationship. So how do we change it? We'll get to that in Part

III, but first, we need to understand why the concept of *healing* is so important to helping solve our healthcare problems.

HEALING JOE

One thing I have learned over the years is that I can never know what to expect when I see a patient for the first time—so I always block off a couple hours. In Joe's case, I used every bit of it.

When I first met Joe, we hit it off pretty quickly, in part because of our mutual friends. Gaining trust is critical with new patients, and I leverage anything I can to obtain it. Once Joe understood I had his best interest at heart, he was willing to share the details of his life.

I started by asking about his family. Understanding a family's medical history allows me to develop a sense of a patient's genetic risk for disease. It's not like sequencing their genome, but it's pretty good—in some ways maybe better, since it tells me what actual diseases they might have caused.

On Joe's father's side, there was a history of severely high cholesterol and depression. On his mother's side, there was a history of stomach problems and strangely enough, fainting. Right away, I knew genetics were at play here. What I needed to know now was how those genes interacted with his environment over the course of his life.

Joe was generally healthy as a kid, but like most of us, his diet consisted of a sugary cereal for breakfast and burgers and fries for lunch. Dinners were described as "meat and potatoes." He rarely ate vegetables. However, he was very successful in sports throughout high school, and he ultimately went to college on a football scholarship and majored in finance.

After college, Joe took a job with an investment banking company. He enjoyed it but found the work stressful, in part due to a demanding boss. He worked long hours, but still maintained an active social life—often going out for beers with friends. Soon thereafter, Joe met his current wife and they married at the age of twenty-five. They would go on to have two daughters over the next five years.

At thirty, Joe started his own business. He enjoyed the independence, but the stress of owning his own business wore on him. Joe worked long hours, juggling his work and family responsibilities. Sleep was optional and he was often tired. Despite the fatigue, he exercised vigorously, usually running five miles, three to five days a week. Exercise was his outlet. Over the years, his diet didn't change much—he still ate a lot of processed foods, especially on the road.

When he was thirty-five, Joe's mother died unexpectedly. This was devastating to the whole family. While they were all able to support one another, Joe struggled. He had been close to his mom. He started having more trouble sleeping and developed feelings of anxiety. His main coping mechanism was exercise, and he became more and more obsessed with it. If he couldn't work out, his whole day would fall apart.

At age forty, Joe saw his primary care physician for a regular medical examination. He was told he was healthy except for elevated cholesterol. It was recommended he take medication, but instead, he continued to focus on exercise over the next ten years.

Then, at age fifty, Joe had his heart attack. Although his blocked artery was fixed, and he was prescribed all the right medications, Joe developed a whole new set of problems—fatigue, brain fog, anxiety, and abdominal pain.

What was going on here? Why did all these new drugs not fix him? From a systems standpoint, it wasn't any particular disease that was the problem. The problem was the litany of environmental stressors that were causing system dysfunction at multiple levels—poor diet, high workload, too much high-intensity exercise, lack of sleep, and high emotional stressors. He was in a constant state of "fight-or-flight" and it affected everything, from his gut function to his blood pressure to his ability to think clearly. The problem wasn't a lack of drugs; the problem was decades of unmitigated stressors.

My prescription for Joe was not more medications or procedures; it was to *simplify* his life to reduce the stressors that were causing system dysfunction in the first place. Of course, changing behavior is hard, but for whatever reason, Joe was ready to make a change. Maybe the two hours I initially spent with him paid off. Or maybe he'd just finally had enough of the pain. Whatever the reason, I took advantage of his willingness to change, and we dug in.

There was a lot Joe needed to change—starting with work. He was able to offload tasks to others and decompress his schedule. He also had to let go of some unhealthy personal relationships. In exchange, he spent more time with his family. I restructured his exercise program to be more balanced with low- and high-intensity aerobics, as well as strength training and stretching. I sent him to a dietician, and we completely overhauled his diet, exchanging bread and pasta for healthy complex carbohydrates with lots of fiber. He also ate more healthy fats and lean protein. He reduced his alcohol use substantially.

And then there was sleep. We used a wearable device to monitor his sleep like a hawk. Joe was a natural early bird, so we picked a sleep window of 9:00 p.m. to 5:00 a.m., and he stuck to it. To facilitate his recovery, I even got him to do some deep breathing and meditation.

So how did things turn out? Over the course of a year, Joe became a *completely different person.* He was happier and healthier than he had been in years. He lost about fifteen pounds. His energy level skyrocketed. His abdominal pain completely resolved, as did his brain fog. In addition, all of his cardiac risk factors improved. His blood pressure dropped. His cholesterol dropped. His blood sugar dropped. Joe was about as far from having another heart attack as he could get.

I didn't do anything "medically" for Joe. No new drugs. No costly procedures. I just sat back and tried to understand what was going on in his life. I had to figure out what was keeping his body from healing and work with him to make a few adjustments. In the end, it wasn't more medicines Joe needed; it was *less stress.*

The problem is that most doctors don't have the time it takes to get to know their patient and figure out all the contributing factors that potentially caused their disease. Insurance doesn't pay for that kind of time. And yet, how much money did Joe cost his insurance company in hospitalizations over the next three years? *Nothing.* How much would another heart attack have cost? *A lot.*

At some point, you'd think insurance companies would figure out how to pay primary care doctors for the invaluable time we spend with our patients—time to get to know them, understand the nuances of their life, and make recommendations on how to improve it. As we will see in Chapter 10, maybe things are changing.

FIXING VERSUS HEALING

Everybody wants a *quick fix*, and everybody expects their doctor to be able to do it. I don't know how many times patients have told me that they simply don't have time to be sick and I need to fix them. *Now.*

Frankly, I love quick fixes too. Imagine this scenario: a young woman comes into my office with a fever and cough. I listen to her lungs and hear the telltale crackles, so I send her to radiology for an X-ray. She has a small pneumonia. I prescribe her an antibiotic, send her on her way, and in a few days, she's feeling better. It's a simple problem with a simple solution.

But nowadays simplicity is the exception. *Complexity is the rule*—multiple symptoms from dysfunction of multiple organs in patients with complex lives is the rule. Reductionism and clinical epidemiology, for all their benefits, are limited in their ability to address these complex conditions.

But this is the essence of systems medicine. As we better understand one's unique genetic makeup and litany of environmental stressors, we could better help patients heal from chronic disease.

But what do we mean by *healing* anyway? And how does it happen? To me, one of the great marvels of biological systems is that they have the innate ability to heal. By healing, I mean a restoration of normal physiological function—and, as a result, elimination of pain and suffering.

Like disease, healing is a process. It's moving from left to right in my graph in Chapter 5. The best part is healing happens naturally. We don't have to *make* it happen. For the most part, we just have to *let* it happen.

We can see healing in action when we accidentally cut ourselves. Immediately, a miraculous series of events takes place. First, little cells called platelets clump together to form a blood clot and stop the bleeding. In fact, a whole cascade of molecules works together to form a clot. Next, the immune system comes in and creates inflammation. This brings in all kinds of cells and molecules to treat infection, debride dead tissue, and send signals to new cells to start the repair process. Next, cells called fibroblasts rush in and produce scar tissue. Finally, a process of tissue remodeling occurs. Remodeling is a long-term process of scar strengthening and restructuring. Over time (upwards of a year), a scar can constantly reform itself in response to small local stressors to form a permanent structure. The whole process happens by itself—if we stay out of the way, of course.[102]

Unfortunately, we are not always good at staying out of the way of the healing process. We pick at our scabs because they irritate us—literally and figuratively. We run on stress fractures because we have to win the race. We work despite having had a heart attack because we have to get that next business deal. We all want to heal from chronic disease, but the reality is, sometimes we cause our own problems.

Let me give you a real-life example of how this works. One of my favorite hobbies was flying gliders with my son Elliot, who was a teenager at the time. Gliders are basically small airplanes with no engine. The idea is you get towed up by a towplane to an altitude of three thousand feet, then you cut yourself loose. You soar around like a bird for as long as you can and then you land on a little grassy runway. You have a stick, rudder pedals, and some instruments to help. *How hard could this be?* I thought.

Flying was actually pretty easy. Landing was sometimes a challenge, but I got that down pretty quickly. But for the life of me, I could not figure out how to hold the glider still behind the towplane while getting towed up. It would go something like this. The glider would slowly drift to the left; I would push the stick right. The glider would go right, then up; I would move the stick down, then left. The glider would go way down and left; I'd get scared and move the stick way up and to the right. Next thing you know, I'd be halfway to the moon and the instructor would have to take over control of the plane. This phenomenon is called *pilot induced oscillations*. In other words, the harder I tried to fix the problem, the worse I made it!

My teenage son, on the other hand, had no problem whatsoever. I asked him what his secret was.

"It's pretty simple, Dad," he said. "I just keep my hand still and use my fingers to make tiny changes in anticipation of the glider's next position."

And there you have it. What I didn't appreciate was that gliders are designed to *self-stabilize*—I just needed to get out of the way. With a little practice, I got pretty good at getting towed up in a glider to three thousand feet, even in some pretty blustery conditions.

The fact is, we often engage in behaviors that contribute to our own dis-ease. Drugs, including alcohol, are the obvious ones, but there are others: work, food, sex, anger, social media, gaming, gambling, shopping, you name it. Everyone has their preferred method to experience pleasure—or at least alleviate discomfort.

So how do we stop causing our own problems? How do we actually change our behavior and let our bodies heal? Like developing any new skill, we need to learn from the experts— those struggling with the disease of addiction.

A NEW WAY OF LIFE

Anthony was in a tough spot. In the thick of his heroin addiction, he found himself living in a cardboard box on a subway grate in downtown Baltimore.

At the time, Anthony was in his late twenties. His life had fallen apart, and he found heroin to be his only coping mechanism. That led to several arrests for possession of drugs, or theft to pay for his drugs. With no home, no friends, and no money, Anthony was living in a constant state of fight-or-flight.

When the drugs stopped working and he couldn't take the pain anymore, Anthony decided to get help. He found a rehab center in the city that agreed to take him as a patient. As they say, *when the pain of staying the same is greater than the pain of changing, we will change.*

I first met Anthony at a twelve-step meeting after he got out of rehab. He was in early recovery, and it was obvious. He was skinny and tired-looking with a large abscess on his forehead. He asked me if I could give him a ride home from the meeting. I told him, "Sure thing, man, but you should probably get that thing looked at first."

He said, "I'll be alright. I get these things all the time." It is amazing how in the midst of immense suffering, us addicts will refuse help. The reality is we don't think we deserve it.

I said, "No, seriously man, hop in my truck and let me take you to an urgent care center."

After he got treatment for what was a serious abscess, I took him home to his father's house. Anthony had stayed with his father in the past but got kicked out after he stole his deceased mother's jewelry for drugs. But Anthony was on a new path now, and his father gave him another chance.

After that night, Anthony showed up to meetings nearly every day. He started working a twelve-step program. He created a new network of other recovering addicts and started *rebuilding* his life. He took responsibility for the problems he created. He showed up in court and cleaned up his legal issues. He worked odd jobs to pay off his debt. Honestly, I'm not sure I ever met someone who worked as hard as Anthony. He was willing to do anything to avoid sleeping on that subway grate in the city.

Today, Anthony is a master plumber. He is married, and he and his wife recently had their first child.

As a result of his hard work, there has been one other blessing bestowed on him: Anthony recently bought a home for him and his family. No more sleeping on a grate. Anthony has found a new way of life.

HEALING FROM ADDICTION

Some people question whether addiction is really a disease. My opinion is this: if we define disease as disordered function of a complex biological system that causes massive pain and suffering, I can assure you that addiction is a disease.

Interestingly, it appears that some people might be genetically predisposed to addiction.[103] Like many diseases, it's possible addiction served as a survival advantage earlier in our evolution.[104] As addicts, we are always looking for something more, something better, something to relieve us of our chronic discomfort—and we will stop at nothing to get it. It used to be food, water, and shelter; now it's alcohol, stimulants, and opiates.

In her book *Dopamine Nation*, Dr. Anna Lembke explains the disease of addiction as a product of the neurotransmitter *dopamine*—a chemical messenger that manages the delicate balance between pleasure and pain. The more dopamine a drug releases into certain parts of our brain, and the faster it releases it, the more addictive the drug.[105] We often start using drugs to alleviate pain—physical or emotional. But many addictive drugs cause *tolerance*—the process by which the body adapts to a drug. Tolerance leads to painful withdrawal symptoms when the drug wears off, creating a drive to pursue more drugs to relieve the pain. It's a vicious cycle of overconsumption, shame, lying, and isolation that some people get trapped in for decades. The only way to start healing from addiction is to get rid of the drugs that started this cycle in the first place. Often that requires getting professional help. Sometimes it requires going to rehab.

When I went to rehab over twenty years ago, I found myself amongst a group of a hundred other struggling addicts. We were all different ages from all walks of life. What we had in common was pain—deep visceral pain from a life that had collapsed within us and around us. No one I met planned on this collapse. In fact, most people got there despite their best efforts not to, including me.

One morning, I was sitting on a bench overlooking the Susquehanna River, thinking about how I got myself into the mess I was in. Out of nowhere, an older man who had recently relapsed on alcohol sat down next to me. Clearly this wasn't his first rodeo. I started telling him how frustrated I was that I could not stop using Ritalin, even though I knew it was destroying me. For the life of me, I could not figure out why I couldn't stop. I mean, I'm a pretty good problem solver, but this one had me stumped.

The man just looked at me and said something I'll never forget. "I understand what you mean. Some of my best thinking created my worst problems." He paused for a moment, then continued, "I've been told you can't think your way into good behaving, but you can behave your way into good thinking."

We talked a little more, then the man just wandered off. Afterward, I sat on my bench and thought about what he said. Then it occurred to me. The solution to my problem was not more thinking; it was more doing. If I wanted to get out of the mess I was in, I needed to make *changes to the way I lived my life*.

Over the years, I have learned there is no fixing addiction. But we addicts can heal from our brokenness and go on to live incredible lives. The process of healing from addiction is called *recovery*. There are many principles I have learned in my own recovery, but three of these have been indispensable, and I believe are instructive in any discussion on healing: *honesty, open-mindedness,* and *willingness*.

Honesty, of course, means not lying. Lying comes easy to many of us. We are often just too ashamed of our behaviors to tell the truth. But honesty means more than not lying to others. It means not lying to ourselves. We need to admit that we have problems in our life—and we had a role in creating those problems. We can't pass all the blame onto others. They say, *when you point the finger at someone else, you have three fingers pointing back at yourself.* Unfortunately, it's true. In order to heal, we have to be honest that we have a role in the problems in our life, and we need to change.

Open-mindedness means being receptive to the idea of changing a behavior; it doesn't mean changing. But most of us don't want to hear it. We'd rather live in a bubble of *confirmation bias*—listening to people who tell us what we *want* to hear rather than what we *need* to hear. Somehow we need to break out of this cycle of self-inflation. In order to heal, we need to be open-minded to suggestions from people who actually care about us, even if we don't want to hear them.

Willingness means making a decision to change a behavior—then changing. Make no mistake about it, letting go of a behavior that relieves us of discomfort is hard, even if we know that behavior is causing us problems in the long run. Sometimes, addictive behaviors are fueled by *resentments*—deep-seated anger for harm that was done to us in the past. But they say, *holding onto resentment is like drinking poison and waiting for the other person to die.* It just doesn't serve a useful purpose. Part of healing, then, involves the willingness to forgive others—then moving forward in a new direction.

I have seen many people heal from chronic disease, including addiction. But the reality is, our healthcare system can't fix, let alone heal, everyone. Sometimes diseases progress. Sometimes people die despite our best efforts. And one of the most important parts of our own healing is letting go.

TOUGH DECISIONS

Harriett was a seventy-seven-year-old, quiet, and unassuming woman, a retired teacher, and the mother of two boys. She was also a lifelong smoker—an addiction she tried unsuccessfully to quit on many occasions.

One thing's for sure, Harriett didn't like talking to doctors, but she would talk to me. Occasionally we would talk about end-of-life situations. Harriett was unambiguous in her desire to not have aggressive measures taken to keep her alive—especially a ventilator, or breathing machine. She had emphysema and knew if she was ever put on a ventilator she would never get off.

Harriett would always say to me, "One day you're just going to give me the needle, aren't you?"

I would always respond by saying, "Well, we don't just give people the needle, but I understand what you are saying." Honoring people's wishes and keeping them from suffering at the end of their life has always been non-negotiable with me.

Harriett was not one to complain about her health. So when she started developing a little abdominal pain, she wasn't really alarmed. But when the pain got bad enough, she finally told her husband and he took her to the local hospital. Initially, it just looked like bad constipation. They decided to admit her for testing.

Harriett must have known something was wrong. As they wheeled her back to her hospital room, she looked at her husband and said, "If I don't make it, I just want you to know it's been a good life." That's a pretty dramatic statement for someone with constipation.

Unfortunately, Harriett went downhill fast. What looked like constipation was actually a *bowel obstruction*—a blocked intestine. This caused vomiting, which caused *aspiration pneumonia*—a condition where things go down the wrong pipe, causing inflammation or infection in the lungs.

Despite her wishes, Harriett was put on a ventilator and admitted to the ICU. Her worst nightmare had come true. Sometimes in the fog of war, people have to make quick decisions, and in this case, everyone was just trying to do the best they could.

The ICU was a closed unit, meaning it had a dedicated doctor, but the ICU doctor allowed me to be part of her care. I helped make decisions and relay information to Harriett's husband and older son. I was mostly a translator, but it was a role with which I had become quite comfortable.

After a couple days in the ICU, things seemed to stabilize. We were cautiously optimistic. Then, her heart started beating irregularly. She developed atrial fibrillation and her blood pressure dropped. This was stabilized with fluids and medications. A temporary fix. Then her kidney function started to deteriorate, as if they were getting tired. That meant giving her more fluids, but the fluid started to leak into her lungs.

It was as if every punch had a counterpunch. The window seemed to be closing. Then, the heart, lungs, and kidneys all seemed to stabilize again. Things seemed to be turning around, and for a moment there was a glimmer of hope.

We decided to wean Harriett off the ventilator, which she never wanted to be on in the first place. The weaning process is as much an art as a science: it's tricky because it's important that a patient be partially conscious so that their own breathing can take over. I was at Harriett's bedside as they started tapering down the sedation, hoping to take her off the ventilator. She started waking up, and I immediately saw the fear in her eyes when she realized she was hooked up to a breathing tube. Then her fear turned to sadness. She could not speak, but with her eyes, I heard her say: *how could you let this happen to me?*

My heart broke. I'll never forget that look she gave me.

Suddenly, Harriett's breathing became more difficult. Her oxygen started to drop. I touched her arm and said, "It's okay. I am right here with you." The nurse turned up the sedation, and she fell back into a deep sleep.

The next morning, there were some tough decisions to make. Harriett couldn't stay in the ICU forever. We had already started talking about transferring her to a long-term care facility on a ventilator—exactly what Harriett did *not* want.

I got there early that morning, as I often do, and hopped on the computer to look at Harriett's numbers. I saw that she had spiked a fever overnight. Also, her heart rate was elevated, and she was back in atrial fibrillation. I looked at her labs. Her electrolytes were off. Her kidney function was deteriorating. Then I saw what would be the final straw. Her white blood cell count was elevated—a sign of a new and serious bacterial infection. In her case, something called *C. difficile colitis*.

Like a tidal wave capsizing a ship, I knew we had lost the battle. There was no way Harriett could survive this infection. After much discussion, her husband made the difficult decision to withdraw care and transfer her to hospice. Harriett died peacefully about eight hours later.

The only good thing about death is that it brings clarity and an end to suffering. At least the roller coaster ride was over and Harriett would not be condemned to a life of hell in a nursing home on a ventilator. After all, there are worse things in life than dying.

I've been in a lot of difficult situations as a physician, but I have to admit, this one was tough. It was also personal. Harriett was not actually a patient of mine—Harriett was my mom.

MOVING ON

At my mother's funeral, I read from 1 Corinthians 13:

> Love is patient, love is kind. It does not envy, it does not boast, it is not proud. It does not dishonor others, it is not self-seeking, it is not easily angered, it keeps no record of wrongs. Love does not delight in evil but rejoices with the truth. It always protects, always trusts, always hopes, always perseveres.

In her quiet and unassuming way, my mother lived these words better than anyone I ever knew. She was the epitome of unconditional love.

When I finished my reading, I looked out at the people gathered there that day and was heartened. What I saw was a community of people who had been touched by my mother's presence in this world. Like recovering addicts, this was a community bonded together, not just by shared pain, but by compassion for one another. I thought for a moment: *Maybe that's what we do at funerals. We come together to help each other heal from the loss of one of our own. We celebrate the life of one of our family and community members. Then we learn to move on without them.*

Complex systems can have complex problems; there is nothing simple about human suffering. Fortunately, we can start to heal from chronic disease if we reduce the stressors that cause it in the first place. But changing behavior is hard. We can't do it alone. We need the help of trained professionals and a confidential place we can go to seek out that help. Primary care should be that place. Primary care lives uniquely at the interface *between* sickness and health; we are in the position to be both fixers *and* healers.

But once healed, then what? Do we just wait until a new problem arises? Are we condemned to repeat cycles of dysfunction, collapse, and regrowth? Or can we prevent dysfunction and collapse from happening in the first place? Maybe we can. But to do that, we need to understand the concept of frailty and think differently about our concept of health.

Let me tell you about a very special patient of mine named Mary.

CHAPTER 8

From Frailty to Health

MARY GREW UP IN BALTIMORE CITY. HER FAMILY WOULD often go days on end without food as her parents waited for the next check to come in. She got pregnant in her teens and married shortly thereafter. She and her husband went on to have two more children together. Unfortunately, as it so often happens with young couples, things got complicated. After eighteen years of marriage Mary and her husband ended up divorcing. That's when things got tough. For years, Mary worked multiple jobs trying to support her kids. They moved from place to place, barely making ends meet. She eventually remarried, and she and her new husband bought a small home. For a while, things were stable.

Then, in her mid-fifties, tragedy struck: her youngest son was killed in a motorcycle accident. Shortly after that she got cancer. She survived the cancer but never really recovered from her son's accident.

For the next several years, Mary got by, but the diseases started piling up—high blood pressure, obesity, diabetes, high cholesterol, osteoporosis, irritable bowel syndrome, depression, anxiety, and knee arthritis. She was put on a litany of medicines to fix each problem, but as the diseases and medications increased, her activity level decreased. Whereas she used to be energetic and active, she became more tired and sedentary. Like many of us, she used food to cope with her discomfort—sugar and carbohydrates in particular. As a result, her weight was increasing, but her strength was decreasing. While she could still function independently, she was getting weaker and weaker.

When I first met Mary, she felt reasonably well and her numbers actually looked pretty good. In particular, her blood pressure, blood sugar, and cholesterol levels were all in the normal range. All the medicines she was taking were working. Her only complaint was severe knee pain.

I obtained X-rays of her knees, which confirmed "bone-on-bone" arthritis, but the arthritis medicine was no longer working. The only solution at this point was a total knee replacement. I referred her to an orthopedic surgery colleague and surgery was scheduled.

Mary's surgery went well, and she was discharged home from the hospital with physical therapy. But things didn't go too well after that. The rehab was harder than she thought. The pain was severe, requiring more pain medications. She got constipated from all the pain medicines, requiring laxatives, which caused diarrhea. Her depression worsened, requiring increases in her antidepressants, which caused more fatigue. If she wasn't getting physical therapy, she would spend most of her time in bed. She was too tired to do anything more. Then one day I got a call from her husband.

"We have a problem," he told me. "Mary just fell coming back from the bathroom. She's back in bed but says she can't do this anymore. She wants out."

What the heck does that mean? I thought.

I went to visit Mary at her home. Her husband greeted me at the door. "She's in the back bedroom," he said.

"Did she hurt herself from the fall?" I asked.

"No," her husband said. "She's okay, she's just done."

I slowly entered her room and softly called her name. When I turned the corner, I found her curled up in bed, crying.

"Mary?" I asked softly. "Are you okay?"

"I just can't take it anymore," she said between sobs. "Every time I get better, something else happens. I can't take it anymore. *I just want to die!*"

I knew Mary well enough to know that she didn't really want to die. Like many of us, she just wanted the pain to go away. I sat down next to her and we talked.

"Mary, I understand how you feel," I said to her. "I really do. But unfortunately, you're not dying. You're just weak from your surgery and all the pain medicines. You can get better. You just have to get stronger. You have to keep going."

Technically, Mary had done everything right. She went into the hospital, had successful surgery, took all of her medications, and was getting home physical therapy. So why was she having so much trouble? Why was everything falling apart?

Mary was frail.

THE FRAILTY SYNDROME

During my fellowship at Hopkins, I had the privilege of working with some of the leaders in geriatrics and frailty research. While my primary interest was sports medicine, the concept of frailty was very interesting to me. As a physical therapist, I saw close up how our strength starts to decline as we age. My older patients were less agile, and their reaction times were slower. As a result, their ability to navigate their environment became more difficult. Tasks that used to be routine—such as shopping, doing laundry, or even getting up and down stairs—became more of a challenge. This would occasionally lead to falls, sometimes with devastating consequences.

About 36 million falls are reported among older adults each year, resulting in more than 32,000 deaths.[106] While some falls are unavoidable, many represent a reduced ability to navigate one's environment. This is often due to a number of problems, including the loss of muscle mass, weakness, reduced endurance, slow walking, and a general decrease in physical activity. These are all components of the frailty syndrome, and they feed on each other to create a cycle of declining human function. It is no surprise that frailty increases the risk of falls, hospitalization, disability, and death.[107]

The study of frailty is also one of the best applications of systems thinking. This is because frailty is not actually a disease: it is the *susceptibility* to disease. It is a state of decreased energy reserves and high vulnerability to environmental stressors. Here's how it goes. As we get older, we lose muscle mass—something called *sarcopenia*. Weaker muscles can't produce as much energy, so people get tired more easily with routine tasks. As people get weaker and more fatigued, they become less active and stress hormones are produced to cope with everyday activities. These stress hormones can cause chronic inflammation and more fatigue. More fatigue causes less activity, and so on in a vicious circle. Over time, a person's whole life starts to contract: physically, mentally, and socially.[108]

In other words, frailty is not due to the decline of any one system. It's due to the cumulative decline of multiple systems, all of which interact with each other at multiple levels—from genes to molecules to cells to organs to the whole person. As a result, the system as a whole loses its ability to regulate itself under stress and eventually crosses a critical threshold—or tipping point.[109]

None of us want to be frail. On the contrary, we want to maintain an active, high-quality life as we age. We want to enjoy our kids and grandkids. We want to travel with our friends. We want to do volunteer work or just live in our own home as long as possible. This is known as *compression of morbidity*—minimizing disease and disability to the smallest amount possible and pushing it to the very end of your life.[110] Dying peacefully in our sleep at a ripe old age after a meaningful life free of disease is most people's idea of compression of morbidity.

So how do we get that deal? How do we live a long life free of chronic disease and recurrent trips to the hospital? First, we need to think differently about health.

Health is the opposite of frailty. It's the ability to navigate all the environmental stressors we discussed in Chapter 6 and somehow press on. Thinking about health in this context pulls us out of our reductionist gaze and toward a systems approach to patient care. We no longer see health merely as the absence of disease—we see it as the *resilience* of a complex biological system.

HEALTH AS RESILIENCE

Resilience is a tricky term, in part because there are so many ways to think about it and in part because it gets complicated really fast. So rather than talk about resilience in any technical way, I'd like to walk you through some real life examples to help you understand how I use the term and how it can be applied to human health.

One way to think about resilience is the ability to avoid injury or illness under high stress conditions. We all know people who experience tremendous adversity, yet press on as if they are walking through fire without flinching. As a physician, I have been with many patients who were under massive amounts of stress, yet when they left my office, the outside world never knew it. They seemed unbreakable, unable to be pushed past a tipping point.

We talked earlier about COVID-19. You may have wondered how some people could walk through a cloud of viral particles and never get sick, yet other people end up on a ventilator, or worse, dying. There are lots of factors that determine whether someone develops a severe illness from COVID-19. Some of it is genetics, some of it is the amount of viral particles they encounter, and some of it is the health of the person who encounters the virus.[111] We learned early on in the pandemic that people with a chronic disease didn't do well with COVID-19. This is likely because chronic disease makes people frail and less resilient, moving them closer to a tipping point. The virus just pushes them over the edge.

Regardless of whether they're exposed to a virus, a chemical toxin, or a demanding job, resilient people seem to *absorb* environmental stressors without getting sick or injured. But everyone has a limit. Even resilient people get sick. In that case, resilience also has something to do with the ability to maintain function in the setting of an injury or illness.

I have worked with many college and professional athletes who had a severe injury yet insisted on getting back on the playing field. Whether they had pulled muscles, sprained ligaments, even broken bones and concussions, some players were always negotiating to get back on the field. But you don't have to be a professional athlete to know resilience in the face of injury or illness. I have known patients to be in the midst of toxic chemotherapy yet never miss a day of work. I have known parents who suffered from severe depression yet still picked their kids up from daycare and made sure they had dinner on the table. Somehow resilient people are able to *compensate* for an injury or illness and keep on going.

Still, sometimes the house of cards really does fall and people need to *reorganize* their lives and rebuild completely. This requires help; no one can rebuild on their own. Recovering from a severe injury or illness requires more than good medical care—it requires a network of family, friends, and other caregivers. Even if you are totally on your own, healing still requires food and shelter. Part of the reason resource scarcity is associated with poor outcomes may be due to the lack of resilience in a patient's ecosystem. In other words, resilience is not just about what's going on *inside* a person; equally important is what's going on *outside*—their network of friends and community resources.

Of course, ideally, we would never get chronic disease or be pushed past a tipping point at all. Resilience might also have something to do with the ability to *adapt* to changing environmental conditions. We talked about adaptation in Chapter 5—bone remodels itself under increasing loads, our brain makes new connections based on new experiences, and our muscle cells get bigger with exercise. By embracing small stressors incrementally, we can adapt to changing conditions over time. In other words, *what doesn't kill us makes us stronger.*

In his book, *What is Health? Allostasis and the Evolution of Human Design*, Peter Sterling describes health as the capacity to respond optimally to fluctuations in demands.[112] And it appears we humans have been dealing with fluctuating demands for thousands of years. As we migrated around the globe, Homo sapiens encountered very harsh conditions, including significant changes in temperature and lack of food. Remarkably, we adapted to these conditions, in part by making small changes to our genes, as we discussed in Chapter 6. But our ability to adapt went beyond the structure of our genes; it also involved the function of our society. According to Sterling, our species learned to *cooperate* in ways that made us much stronger as a group. In a group, one person's strengths could overcome another person's weakness. Together, we had all bases covered. It appears being genetically unique and cooperating as a group has made us a resilient species indeed.

So if we define health as resilience, it begs the question: *Are there things we can do to improve our health and avoid frailty as we age? Can we strategically plan for unforeseen stressors and adapt ahead of time?* The answer is, emphatically, *yes*! Health does not come only from taking medications, it comes from making changes to the way we live our lives.

Over the years, I have provided recommendations to my patients on how they can improve their health, and I would like to share them with you. If you are not interested in making changes to your life, I understand. Change is hard. You are more than welcome to skip ahead to Chapter 9. After all, there are plenty of drugs and hospitals out there to treat you when you get sick. But if you are interested, let's take a more detailed look at how you can improve your health and possibly avoid the sickcare system altogether.

EXERCISE: TRAIN FOR THE FUTURE YOU

Let's face it, navigating our environment becomes more and more difficult as we age. At an advanced age, that environment can even become our own home! In order to help my patients avoid injury and maintain a high quality of life as they age, I want them to remain independent with *Activities of Daily*

Living (ADLs)—the set of activities we all engage in on a daily basis. By independent, I mean that they can perform these tasks without the assistance of another person.

I learned about ADLs as a physical therapist, and I still use them in my primary care practice thirty years later. At the very least, I want my older patients to remain independent with *Basic ADLs*—activities required for self-care, such as getting in and out of bed, walking short distances, using the bathroom, and eating. Ideally, I want them to be able to perform *Instrumental ADLs*—activities required for independent living, such as shopping, cooking, dressing, and managing finances.

While all these tasks are important, my real goal for patients is higher than Basic or Instrumental ADLs. I want patients to be engaged in whatever activities are important to them—gardening, dancing, hiking, camping, volunteer work, traveling, recreational sports, or just playing with their grandchildren. I call these *Advanced ADLs,* and to me, they are the essence of a meaningful life.[113]

Of course we don't want to wait until something bad happens—like a fall or a stroke—before we start worrying about ADLs. If we want to stay active and avoid the sickcare system altogether, we need to start training now! This means we need to *exercise*—intentionally challenging ourselves physically, cognitively, and socially—so we can improve our resilience and fend off any stressors that might come our way down the road. Let's discuss all three of these, starting with physical exercise.

There are many ways to think about physical exercise, but I'd like to share a framework I developed based on my training and experience over the years. I break exercise down into five general categories of increasing complexity: mobility and stability exercises, low intensity exercise, resistance training, high intensity interval training, and functional training. The types and amount of exercise you engage in depends on your state of health and personal goals. As such, you should always seek the advice of a medical provider, physical therapist, or certified trainer prior to exercise. With that said, let me share how I discuss exercise with my patients—and how I exercise myself.

Mobility and stability are two sides of the same coin. They work together to help us move through our environment in a smooth and efficient manner. Some of us have problems with mobility even at a young age—often from previous injuries. Left unaddressed, they only get worse over time. Ever see an older person hunched over a walker? That is due to loss of mobility of the upper spine, but it could be prevented by doing postural exercises early in life. In a related way, stability exercises are designed to maintain our balance as we move from one position to another, such as with lifting, squatting, or walking. Maintaining good balance is critical to navigating our environment and preventing falls as we age.

After addressing issues with movement, I discuss low intensity exercise or endurance training. This could include a brisk walk, riding a stationary bike, or using one of many types of exercise equipment for a longer duration, such as a half hour or more. And by low intensity, I mean exercising as hard as we can while still being able to carry on a conversation. (Hint—it's not very intense.) The value of low intensity exercise cannot be overstated. When we engage in this type of exercise, we are training our body to burn fat for energy.[114] Fat is burned inside *mitochondria*—small structures inside cells where the vast majority of energy is made from the food we eat. By training our muscles to burn fat, we are training them to improve mitochondrial function.[115] And improving mitochondrial function can reduce our risk of insulin resistance and diabetes.[116]

After low intensity exercise, I discuss *resistance training*—pushing, pulling, and lifting against some type of resistance like dumbbells, rubber bands, or just our own body weight. Make no mistake about it, building and maintaining muscle tissue as we age is *critical* if we want to avoid sarcopenia and the frailty syndrome we discussed earlier.[117] Resistance training has other benefits as well. It reduces body fat and the risk of diabetes, improves cardiovascular health, reduces blood pressure and cholesterol, increases bone density, improves mental health, and maybe slows the aging process itself.[118] Increasing muscle tissue by resistance training is also a good example of adaptation. When we lift heavy objects such as a dumbbell, the body adapts in preparation for lifting more heavy objects. It does this by activating genes that make muscle from the protein we eat.[119] As a result, we get stronger over time.

After strength training I discuss *high intensity interval training*—brief intervals of exercise such as running, cycling, or rowing at a faster pace. These intervals are designed to burn carbohydrates for energy, and they can improve our metabolic rate, insulin sensitivity, and cognitive function.[120] High intensity exercises also improve our *metabolic flexibility*—the ability to go back and forth between burning carbohydrates and fat for energy. Being metabolically flexible could help prevent or treat chronic diseases such as obesity, diabetes, cardiovascular disease, chronic inflammation, and even cancer.[121] But we have to be a little careful here. Too much high intensity exercise can be a stressor and cause an injury or even an acute illness.

After developing a foundation of fitness based on all the activities above, I discuss *functional training*—more dynamic activities performed in a complex environment, often with other people. As such, they are often great social activities. These activities focus on balance, coordination, and agility and can be performed at low or high levels of intensity. They might include functional fitness classes, martial arts, and competitive sports. Or they might include ballet or ballroom dancing. For me, the main benefit of functional training isn't so much about health, but *performance*. It is the best way to prepare physically for any serious or life-threatening situation that might come my way—such as surviving a severe storm or escaping a burning building. Remember that word resilience? This is part of what I was talking about.

But beyond good physical function, if we want to stay resilient as we age, we need good cognitive function as well. We need a good memory and the ability to think clearly and rationally. Fortunately, one of the best ways to maintain or improve cognitive function is with physical exercise.[122] But cognitive exercises can also help. Many of us get our fill of cognitive exercise with school or work, but other activities—such as reading, writing, crossword puzzles, board or card games, group discussions, or playing music—have been shown to improve cognitive function as well.[123] Combining physical and cognitive activities is even better.[124] Nonetheless, patients still ask me all the time: *isn't there a pill you can give me to improve my memory?* Sorry to say, despite what you might hear from your friends, it's not that simple. If you want to improve your memory and cognitive function, you need to live a healthy lifestyle.

Finally, on top of physical and cognitive exercise, it turns out that healthy social relationships can also help improve our resilience.[125] We humans are social creatures. As we discussed earlier, our ability to cooperate with one another is a large reason we survived as a species. It makes sense then, if we want to live a long meaningful life, we need to develop healthy relationships.

While we often talk about physical and cognitive exercise, we don't really talk about social exercise, but we probably should. For some of us, being a better person takes practice no different than being a better athlete. I learned this lesson the hard way—in rehab. One way to develop healthy relationships is by being an active member of a community. Communities are networks of people that emerge in society based on shared values, beliefs, and interests.[126] There are many different types of communities we can belong to. For example, I am part of a recovery community, farming community, fitness community, and medical community. When I need help I reach out to one of my friends, and when they need help they reach out to me. We all have unique skill sets, and together, we have all bases covered. Make no mistake about it, I believe having a strong network of friends *now* will improve my ability to manage unforeseen stressors down the road.

Engaging in regular physical, cognitive, and social activities can help us remain healthy and resilient for years to come. But it takes energy to do all this. To get the maximal benefit from these activities, we need to follow it up with good nutrition and adequate recovery. Let's start with nutrition.

NUTRITION: EAT WHAT YOU NEED, NOT WHAT YOU WANT

When I discuss nutrition with my patients, I start with what the body needs. Like exercise, everyone is unique, and even one person's needs can change depending on their activity level and goals. For patients with nutritional-related diseases, like obesity and diabetes, I recommend seeing a registered dietitian for formal advice. But for the average person looking to stay healthy, I focus on three aspects of nutrition: *macro*nutrients, *micro*nutrients, and meal timing.

When I talk about macronutrients, I'm talking about sources of *calories*—energy to do work like ADLs or exercise. Macronutrients are fuel; they primarily consist of carbohydrates and fats. Let's start with carbs.

Carbohydrates get a lot of attention these days, for good reason. Carbohydrates are sugar molecules linked together like boxcars on a freight train. *Simple* or refined carbohydrates have a few sugar molecules linked together. *Complex* carbohydrates have a lot of sugar molecules linked together. Why is this important? The more complex the carbohydrate, the longer it takes the body to digest it, or break it down, and the slower it is absorbed into your bloodstream. This helps prevent metabolic diseases like diabetes and heart disease. Complex carbohydrates are a healthy source of fuel for the body and they can be found in all kinds of vegetables, fruits, whole grains, berries, and beans.[127]

One particular type of complex carbohydrate is fiber. Increasing natural fiber intake has been shown to have many health benefits, including improved weight loss; lower blood pressure, serum cholesterol, and blood sugar levels; improvements in gastroesophageal reflux disease, constipation, and hemorrhoids; and enhanced immune function.[128] When I consider my own nutrition, I make a point of eating high-fiber foods, including whole grains, fruits, vegetables, berries, and beans.

Fats get a lot of attention these days too. One of the greatest sources of confusion over the past several decades has been whether fat is good or bad for you. At this point in time, most experts agree that *unsaturated fats* from whole foods—such as olives, avocados, nuts, seeds, and fish—are probably good for you.[129] What seems to get everybody's blood boiling are *saturated fats*—fats primarily from animal products. Personally, I suspect this falls into the "no one-size-fits-all" category. For some people, saturated fats seem to raise LDL cholesterol levels and may increase the risk of heart disease.[130] I have also seen this firsthand. However, in other people it doesn't seem to make much of a difference. The bigger issue, in my opinion, is the source of fat. Fats should come from natural whole foods, not manufactured from some refinery.

Another macronutrient is protein. Dietary protein is not used so much for energy as it is building blocks for the body to make its own protein, such as muscle or other types of connective tissue. Protein is made from individual *amino acids* that are linked together similar to carbohydrates. When we eat protein, it is broken down into these amino acids and absorbed into our bloodstream. Our cells can then reassemble these amino acids to make whatever type of protein our body needs. How much protein should we eat every day? Probably more than we think.[131] Eating protein is critical if we want to maintain muscle mass as we age and avoid the frailty syndrome. Sources of protein include chicken, fish, beef, and eggs, but plants offer an excellent source of protein as well, especially beans, nuts, and many whole grains.[132]

Micronutrients are basically vitamins, minerals, and trace elements. They often serve as cofactors for *enzymes*—specialized protein molecules that regulate biochemical reactions that are critical for normal cellular function. We can ensure adequate micronutrients by eating a variety of healthy, colorful foods. What are these? They are the same foods we discussed above—fruits, vegetables, whole grains, nuts, seeds, berries, beans, and healthy sources of protein. If you do not eat a lot of these foods, taking a high-quality multivitamin might not be a bad idea.[133]

It's one thing to talk about *what* to eat. But how about *when* to eat? There's a lot of buzz out there these days about *intermittent fasting*—structured periods of time when you are not eating any calories, say from 7:00 p.m. until 7:00 a.m. the next day. Fasting has been part of human civilization forever and appears to have some health benefits.[134] Why would fasting improve your health? At the very least, it helps us eat fewer calories, which helps with diseases such as obesity and diabetes.[135] It might also help our gut microbiome.[136] But one benefit of fasting might be what happens at a cellular level. With more prolonged fasts, our cells undergo a process called *autophagy*—a dynamic recycling process that produces new building blocks and energy for cellular renovation and homeostasis.[137] In other words, cells can deconstruct themselves during a fasted state and reconstruct themselves during a fed state. Creation, destruction, re-creation. That sounds familiar. It turns out autophagy might be a mechanism cells use to adapt to high-stress conditions.[138]

So those are the nutrients you *need.* But what is it that you really *want?* I don't know about you, but I want bread, pasta, pretzels, chips, and ice cream. And while these might be perfectly fine if consumed in moderation, I don't do anything in moderation. For an addict like me, *one is too many and a thousand is never enough!* Anybody who has ever eaten an entire bag of potato chips knows what I'm talking about. We all crave things that give us pleasure or relieve us of discomfort—and food is a big one. To manage cravings, I try to be aware of them and what might be driving them. In recovery, we often use the acronym *HALT*—hungry, angry, lonely, and tired. It does seem that my cravings are worse when I feel tired and frustrated. Part of managing my cravings, then, is getting adequate sleep and creating a temporary reprieve from daily stressors. Let's discuss them next.

RECOVERY: LET THE TIDE GO OUT

We all need to recover from a full day of activity, and that starts with a good night's sleep. However, while I might have learned a lot about exercise and nutrition prior to my medical training, I learned nothing about sleep. For that matter, I learned little about sleep during my medical training. All I learned was that needing sleep meant you were weak. It's probably no surprise, then, that I fell in love with a drug that could keep me awake.

I have to admit my bias here. *I believe sleep is one of the most underappreciated activities to improve our health.* Much of that comes from my own experience, but there are more and more studies to support this notion. In his book, *Why We Sleep*, Matthew Walker explains in detail the detriments of lack of sleep—worse attention and concentration; less emotional control and impulsive behaviors; increased incidence of chronic disease such as obesity, diabetes, and heart disease; immune system dysfunction; reduced athletic performance; and even earlier death.[139] Not surprisingly, getting adequate sleep improves your memory and motor task efficiency. It also helps clear out harmful metabolic waste products, including proteins associated with Alzheimer's Disease.

But just as it's not as easy as telling people to start exercising, it's not as easy as just telling people to get more sleep. In modern society, we have a multitude of stressors getting in the way of our natural sleep-wake cycles, or circadian rhythms. But the better we can tap into our circadian rhythms and get a good night's sleep, the better we can recover from our previous day's activities. Based on the work of Dr. Walker and others, here are some pointers I give to my patients and follow myself to help get a good night's sleep:

First, keep your bedroom dark, quiet, and cool—around sixty-five degrees. A drop in core body temperature is one of the biggest triggers for sleep. Second, reduce or avoid excess food, alcohol, and caffeinated beverages prior to bed. Nothing wrecks my sleep more than eating a big meal right before bed. Of course, I realize that many of our social activities occur at night, so I suggest making late-night dinners the exception rather than the rule. Third, try to minimize watching TV, checking your phone, or working on your computer after dark. If you do, wear glasses that block the blue light that suppresses the sleep hormone melatonin. Fourth, avoid high intensity activities late in the evening. Instead, engage in relaxing activities that quiet your fight-or-flight response. Finally, if you still have trouble getting to sleep, get a sleep study. Sleep apnea is a significant cause of poor sleep and poor health.

But we don't need to wait until nighttime to take a break from the madness. It can be just as powerful to create our own reprieve from stressors of the day—be it resting from strenuous activity, taking a relaxing walk, or maybe trying some meditation. Personally, I never really understood meditation. As someone with a brain that never shuts off, the idea of sitting still and not thinking was simply a foreign concept. But I was always envious of people who could meditate; they seemed to have a tool they could use to relieve the daily stressors of life. So I learned something about it. Let me share one such experience.

Once, in the middle of a hectic workday, I was getting frustrated and knew I needed to take a break. I decided to try meditating. I sat still and tried to let my mind go blank. I took a deep breath in and slowly let it out. But various thoughts came crashing into my head. It reminded me of watching my sandcastle get pounded by the waves as a kid.

I thought of how crashing waves as a kid are like telephone calls, text messages, and emails as an adult. Both involve feelings of being overwhelmed and unable to keep up with the onslaught. As a kid, I would eventually give up and go back to my beach house. But I thought to myself, *What would have happened if I had just stayed at the beach?* I imagined more waves, more foam, more energy, more turbulence. I just sat there in my mind, watching my sandcastle get completely consumed by the ocean.

As I continued meditating, the waves eventually started to die down. Slowly, they got smaller and smaller and further out to sea until they were nothing but tiny ebbs and flows lapping the shoreline. The tide had gone out. I thought to myself, *When exactly is low tide anyway? How can you tell exactly when low tide ends and high tide begins?* As I pondered these questions, it felt as if time stood still. I found myself caught somewhere between the past and the future, all the while enjoying the stillness of low tide.

Suddenly, there was a knock at my door. It was my assistant letting me know my next patient was here. It was time to get back to work. I thought to myself, *I guess the tide is starting to come back in.* I smiled and went out to greet my next patient.

I'm not sure if that qualifies as meditation, but it was an interesting experience. Since then, I have learned to create similar experiences. In the midst of chaos, I will take a deep breath in and slowly let it back out. And in between breaths, I enjoy the peace of low tide.

Engaging in regular physical, cognitive, and social activities, nourishing yourself with healthy foods, and allowing time to recover can help your body become more resilient. But something else seems to happen to my patients as they become healthier: sometimes their entire sense of well-being changes. Sometimes, they even find new meaning to their lives.

A NEW PURPOSE

You might have been asking yourself, *whatever happened to Mary anyway?* Well, after we got through that difficult day, Mary made a commitment to getting her strength back. We tapered her off her pain medications, and she worked hard with physical therapy. Yes, she still had pain, but she didn't let it stop her. She started doing more work around the house, making her more active. She also started eating better. And of course, she slept. Over time, she got stronger, and her pain eventually subsided.

Mary had a setback when her husband died unexpectedly. They were inseparable and committed to each other in their own way. But by this point, Mary was no longer frail; she was resilient. So she kept moving forward.

Today Mary is doing well. She moved into a retirement community and spends most of her time with her children, grandchildren, and a few close friends. She is actively involved in her church and has even helped comfort babies in withdrawal born to women who are opiate addicts. Mary has a gift for loving and caring for others, and she uses it to make the world around her a better place. Is Mary's life different now? Of course it is. She has found a new purpose.

You have a purpose in life too. Since you have a unique set of genes and life experiences, you have something to offer this world that no one else can offer. Sure, maybe it's something big like starting a nonprofit or working at a local homeless shelter, but it doesn't have to be. Maybe it's just holding the door open for someone at a convenience store. Or leaving a nice tip for a struggling waitress. Or asking an older person on an elevator how their day is going. Every day, you have an opportunity to make a positive impact on another person. You just need to make a decision to do it.

In order to have your biggest impact in this world, though, you need to be healthy. Of course, primary care *should* be the place you go to get healthy, but right now, primary care is still broken. It is handcuffed by high patient volume and administrative complexity. If we really want to improve people's health, we need to reinvent the primary care model. After that, we need to make it the foundation of a new American healthcare system. Only then will we truly reduce the burden of chronic disease and avoidable hospitalizations in this country. I believe it's possible—we just need to reorganize a few things and start *rebuilding*.

Part III will show us how to do exactly that. It will show how we could combine a systems-based *clinical* model and a value-based *financial* model to create a truly coordinated healthcare system. With any luck, by the end of the next two chapters, everything will make sense. Then we'll talk about putting our words into action.

We'll start Part III by exploring the foundation of a new primary care model: the physician-patient relationship and my experience with a young man named Derek.

The Future of Medicine

CHAPTER 9

Reinventing Primary Care

DEREK WAS A YOUNG MAN IN HIS EARLY TWENTIES—NOT
much younger than I was when I met him during my internship at The Johns Hopkins Hospital. While I would see Derek
in the hospital when he was admitted to our service, I also
became his primary care doctor at the local community health
center.

Derek was raised by his mother. It was just the two of them, as
his father moved to a different city after he was born, and he
had no siblings. Just after turning one year old, Derek developed an *intussusception*—a condition where the small intestine
"telescopes" inside itself, causing an obstruction, or blockage, of
the bowel. His situation was complicated by a severe infection
requiring emergency surgery. Although he survived and recovered, he was left with a large scar and recurrent abdominal pain.

Life was tough for Derek—growing up on the streets of Baltimore without a father wasn't easy. He was a good kid, but he struggled in high school and dropped out after getting a girl pregnant. He worked a series of odd jobs, but without a high school diploma, he couldn't find anything permanent.

I first met Derek when he was admitted to Hopkins for recurrent abdominal pain. He had never been to Hopkins before and I was a new intern, so I was determined to make the diagnosis and impress my senior resident—but after an extensive work-up, I could find no definitive cause of his pain. Eventually he just got better and was discharged home.

Derek was admitted three times over the next three months with the same complaints. While I was able to control his pain with medications, I was never able to come up with a diagnosis. I decided I had to deal with this when I saw him at the community health center.

On the day I was to see Derek, I confided in one of the clinic's social workers, named Dan, about how frustrated I was that Derek kept coming back to the hospital with abdominal pain. I was getting to the point where I just didn't believe him. Dan gave me the best advice anyone could give a young primary care doctor in training.

"Just talk to him and see what's going on in his life," he told me. "Get to know him a bit."

That sounded great, but forming a relationship with a patient in a community health center was a challenge on two fronts. First, there was no time. We had about thirty minutes per patient, including paperwork—and even that was a luxury. Most staff physicians had half that amount of time. But I convinced my administrator to let me have extra time with Derek and bought myself an hour.

The second challenge was more problematic. Here I was, a kid from the suburbs of Philadelphia, trying to connect with a kid from the streets of East Baltimore. I needed some way to connect with Derek. I needed him to trust me. But what did we have in common? We were from two different worlds.

At least we were about the same age and we were both men, I thought. *Maybe that would give me some credibility.* Then it occurred to me, *We were also both fathers of little girls.* In fact, it turned out our girls were about the same age. I decided to give it a shot.

When I walked into the exam room, I found Derek sitting hunched forward on a chair next to a small desk. He wasn't a big guy, but the exam rooms in community health centers are not big either. You are practically on top of each other.

I sat down at the desk with Derek sitting to my right. We were eye to eye. To break the ice, I did what my friend Dan told me to do: I just started talking with him. I asked him how things were going, where he lived, and how his daughter was doing. Then I asked him what it was like growing up in East Baltimore. I wanted to understand the obstacles he faced in his life—obstacles I could never appreciate. Interestingly, over the course of the conversation, I started to feel a connection with Derek. There was no doubt that being fathers to little girls created a bond between us. But there was something else going on—I just wasn't sure what it was.

That day was the beginning of a long process. For the next two and a half years, I would see Derek off and on at the health center and also in the hospital, where he would continue to show up with abdominal pain. When I did see him, I would do some of the normal doctor things—examine him, check some labs, and treat his pain—but mostly we just talked.

Over time, I learned a couple important things. First, Derek loved his little girl. He was a good father. Second, his relationship with his girlfriend was complex and emotionally charged.

Then I noticed a pattern. Most of the pain crises Derek experienced were preceded by an argument with his girlfriend. When Derek said he was in pain, he wasn't lying—I believe he felt abdominal *pain*. It just wasn't an abdominal *disease* that was causing his pain. It was a tidal wave of psychological and emotional trauma that came back to haunt him.

Even though I developed a connection with Derek, that didn't mean it was the easiest doctor-patient relationship. Derek was charismatic and a bit of a sweet-talker. There were many times I thought he was just bullshitting me to get more pain meds.

Over the next couple of years, I would work with Dan to get Derek whatever services I could—medical services, family counseling, financial support, and so on. Derek would do well for a while, but he would still occasionally show up in the ER with abdominal pain.

On my last day of residency, I was finishing up some paperwork when I was paged. It was Derek calling, complaining of abdominal pain and begging for more pain medicine. As we spoke on the phone, I felt like I was being played. It felt like all the time I had spent trying to connect with him and help him was for naught.

"Listen Derek, I've finished my residency," I told him. "I can't prescribe pain medicines for you anymore. You have a new doctor now. You have to call them from here forward."

When he pushed back and started laying a guilt trip on me, I uncharacteristically let him have it.

"You know, Derek, you're so much better than this," I said. "What are you going to do, just bounce from doctor to doctor looking for pain meds every time you get into a fight with your girlfriend? You have a lot to offer this world, but you don't see it."

He lashed back at me. "You just don't understand!" he yelled. "You don't know what it's like!"

"You're right, Derek. I don't know what it's like! But what I do know is you have a little girl and she deserves to have a father who can be there for her. For her sake, I hope you can figure this out."

With that I hung up the phone, my hand shaking from the anger of being played one more time.

Little did I know it then, but I would go on to have my own issues with prescription drugs a few years later. In hindsight, maybe that was the deeper connection I felt with Derek. We were both struggling young men who would turn to prescription drugs to deal with our pain. Only I had the resources to move onto a path of recovery. And him? I guess his obstacles were too difficult to overcome.

After my residency, I moved on to my fellowship and honestly forgot about Derek. In the end, he was just one of thousands of patients I would see over my ten years of medical training in Baltimore City.

Several years later, things were going pretty well for me. I was in an active recovery program, remarried, raising my kids, and enjoying a successful practice.

One day, my wife, Karen, and I went to an outdoor concert with some friends. We were walking around the large crowd in front of the stadium when I suddenly heard someone call out, "Doctor Queale! Doctor Queale!"

I stopped dead in my tracks. My heart sank. I knew that voice.

Holy shit, I thought. *It's Derek.*

I turned around and standing there in front of me was a strapping, well-dressed young man. I almost didn't recognize him.

"Derek?" I asked.

"Yeah, it's me!"

I walked up to him and gave him a big hug.

"Derek, you look great," I said. "How are you doing? What's going on with you these days?"

"I'm doing great, Doc," he said. "Things are going really well. I ended up getting my GED and a degree from a local community college. Now I have a great job working for a company in Washington, DC."

"That's fantastic," I said.

Then I asked him about his abdominal pain.

"It's gone, Doc," he replied. "I don't need pain meds anymore. My girlfriend and I worked through some stuff, and everything is good now."

"And how's your little girl?"

"She's great. She's a teenager now and we're close. Real close."

Then he said something that I'll never forget.

"Doc, I really want to thank you for what you said to me that last day we talked."

"Derek," I said sheepishly, "I don't think I *said* anything. I think I just yelled at you. I'm really sorry about that."

"It's okay, Doc. You said what I needed to hear, and I just wanted to say thanks."

We chatted a bit more, gave each other another hug, and moved on.

Being a physician is hard. But every once in a while, you make a connection with a patient that makes it all worth it.

THE PHYSICIAN-PATIENT RELATIONSHIP

My experience with Derek speaks to the foundational principle of primary care—the physician-patient relationship. Without a trusting relationship with my patient, the likelihood of them taking their medicine or making a lifestyle change is slim to none. Yet, as we have already seen, most primary care physicians don't have the time to develop a relationship with their patients. They have too many patients on their schedule or are too consumed with administrative work. If we are to truly reinvent primary care, we need to envision a future in which primary care physicians have the time, and resources, to make meaningful connections with their patients.

However, it's not just about time. It's also important to create an environment where patients feel they can be honest and won't be judged negatively for their past failures. Healing, as we discussed, starts with honesty. If my office is not a confidential environment where people can share what's truly troubling them, then all they will do is bury their troubles deep down and live with resentment and fear, which will only express itself as chronic disease somewhere down the road.

Some would argue that this intensive relationship building isn't the role of primary care, that it should fall under the jurisdiction of a licensed therapist or psychiatrist. But a psychiatry colleague once told me, "Nobody is in a better position to do supportive therapy for patients than a primary care doctor." In reality, behavioral health should be integrated into primary care, and there are efforts to do so.[140] But all we really need is time with our patients—time to get to know them and help them navigate a complex situation. If there is a serious mental illness going on, we can refer them to a psychiatrist for a further evaluation and treatment.

The physician-patient relationship is critical to delivering effective primary care. But simply getting in to see a primary care doctor isn't all that easy. In fact, a recent study found the average wait time to see a family medicine doctor was twenty-nine days in large markets and fifty-four days in mid-sized markets![141] That begs the question, *Are there ways we can improve access to primary care? Does it always have to be a physician?* Maybe not. Let's explore some of the options.

PRIMARY CARE IS A TEAM EFFORT

While I love the concierge model for the amount of time it provides with my patients, it suffers from a major flaw: it creates the expectation that I can do everything myself. This might have worked well in the early days, when the administrative aspect of medicine was more simple, but it does not work in today's complex environment—not even in a concierge model. Nowadays, primary care is a team effort. By team I mean an expansive group of providers and administrative personnel, often from different organizations.

And while I often use the term primary care *physician*, it's important to point out that a physician doesn't always have to be the primary point of contact for a patient. In fact, other providers—such as nurse practitioners (NPs) and physician assistants (PAs)—are perfectly well suited, sometimes even better suited, to establish a trusting relationship with patients. We talked about nurse practitioners earlier. Physician assistants work in a similar fashion, usually under some type of supervision by a physician. NPs and PAs are often seen as filling the gap caused by a growing shortage of primary care physicians in this country, especially in rural areas.[142]

Unfortunately, right now NPs and PAs are often seen as a mechanism to increase volume of care rather than quality of care. Remember Erin's story from Chapter 3? She was dumped on by overworked and burnt-out physicians. That model simply doesn't work. If NPs and PAs are going to develop trusting and effective relationships with their own patients, they need time and administrative support just like their physician colleagues.

Beyond NPs and PAs, there are many other potential members of a primary care team, including registered nurses, social workers, behavioral health specialists, dietitians, physical therapists, and pharmacists. Equally as important are the administrative personnel who do an enormous amount of work behind the scenes—scheduling patients; managing electronic medical record systems; dealing with insurance companies; managing prescription refills; and coordinating labs, tests, consultations, and hospital admissions. And since primary care offices are members of their local community, the administrative team often knows all the local community resources, such as housing, transportation services, substance abuse programs, food banks, and other social support services. Make no mistake about it, effective primary care really is a team effort.[143]

But it's not just medical providers that help our patients. On the other end of the provider spectrum—and very much a part of the primary care team—are patients' family members. It turns out there are about 53 million family and friends providing care and assistance to loved ones in the United States, yet they are often overlooked by our healthcare system.[144] Family members can provide significant insight and assistance to a patient's primary care team—insight and assistance that cannot be obtained in any comparable fashion.

How do we link these two teams together? Who serves as the bridge between the providers in the office and the providers in the home? In the community health program we discussed, the primary point of contact with a patient was not even a medical provider; it was a community health worker—a person without any prior medical experience whatsoever. What they did have was a desire to help people and an innate ability to connect at a deep and authentic level. The reason our program was so successful was because of the trusting relationship they developed with their patient and their savviness in breaking down barriers to effective care.

While community health workers are often deployed in disadvantaged communities, they could have applications in any community. A new workforce of *community healthcare providers*—be they community health workers, health coaches, or even emergency medical technicians—could expand the reach of primary care physicians outside the office and into *all* the communities they serve.[145] This new workforce could provide care to patients who often have no alternative but to dial 911 after they get pushed past a tipping point.

However, out in front of a workforce of community-based

healthcare providers lies another potential source of help for primary care—*technology*. And I'm not talking about telemedicine; that's just a video version of an office visit. I'm talking about *automated care*—primary care services that are offered to patients by computer algorithms under the guidance of a primary care physician.

While it might seem counterintuitive, it turns out patients often feel more comfortable confiding in a computer than an actual person.[146] Regardless of such value, automated primary care platforms could be a game changer to the extent they can provide a low-cost alternative to human caregivers. In this way, they could enhance efficiency and clinical quality while freeing physicians to spend more time with patients who need it most.[147] But these platforms would not exist in isolation or be relegated to consumers; they would be a critical component of a new primary care *system*.

The integration of office-based, community-based, and technology-based care could create a spectrum of access points for all members of a local community. The access point could be determined by the level of medical complexity and the choice of the patient. The important point is that patients would have a connection to a primary care *system* that includes people who care about them—a system that provides a confidential setting where they could be honest and receive medical care with empathy and compassion and without judgment. Such a system could provide rapid access to high-quality primary care services for all members of a community at a lower cost. If that's not value-based care, I don't know what is.

Of course, once a patient has access to a new primary care

system, it's time to get to work. What do primary care providers do in this new system? What does a primary care model based on systems medicine look like? Let's take a look.

PREVENTION, EARLY DETECTION, AND MITIGATION

They say *an ounce of prevention is worth a pound of cure.* That begs the question, *Can we really prevent disease from occurring in our patients?* I made the argument in Chapter 6 that we need to rethink chronic disease as disordered function of a complex system due to a genetic predisposition and a litany of environmental stressors encountered on a daily basis. Furthermore, I made the argument in Chapter 8 that an individual's resilience can be improved by engaging in physical, cognitive, and social activities, proper nutrition, and adequate recovery. I believe both approaches—reducing excessive environmental stressors and improving system resilience—can help prevent disease.

Prevention is by far the best medicine. But from a practical standpoint, prevention isn't always possible. We simply cannot identify all contributing factors that lead to disease, and few people have the resources or discipline to significantly improve their resilience. As a result, disease will happen despite our best efforts.

The next best thing, then, is *early detection and mitigation*— detecting disease as early as possible and intervening to minimize progression or restore normal function. What do I mean by that? Ideally, it's reducing the stressors that caused disease in the first place—smoking, poor diet, an unhealthy relationship, and so on—or possibly curing it with medications or surgery. Regardless of how we approach it, the sooner we can catch a disease the better. After all, it's easier to put out a campfire than a forest fire.

So what is early detection in today's medicine? Good examples are what we call *age-appropriate screening*—blood pressure checks, mammograms, colonoscopies, and various lab tests such as a prostate-specific antigen, or PSA. Newer tests can even detect tiny bits of cancer DNA in the blood to catch cancers very early in the process, and these "liquid biopsies" have significant potential.[148]

The truth is, relative to what the future holds, these are still pretty crude. They still detect disease *after* it happens. But advances in technology are likely to revolutionize the way we look at early detection. And these advances might allow us to detect dysfunction so early in the process that we can intervene before a disease—at least the way we currently think about it—ever develops. In effect, early detection and mitigation become a form of prevention!

One major technological advance will come in the form of the advanced sensors and computer modeling we discussed earlier. When you look at disease as system dysfunction, you can start to imagine how we could use the same principles that engineers use to detect instability in an airplane or a spacecraft to detect instability in the human body at a physiological, cellular, or even molecular level. These systems would have sensors that collect and send data to Artificial Intelligence (AI) algorithms, which would allow adjustments to be made to restore normal function. But this is more than just theory. Early warning systems are already appearing in intensive care units, where severe drops in blood pressure can be identified an hour before they actually happen.[149]

One of the best applications of early detection technology might be in a patient's own home. New *Smart Medical Homes* could provide continuous interaction with patients in real time—receiving information through advanced sensors to feed AI algorithms.[150] These algorithms could replicate the expertise of physicians without really going beyond what a physician currently does in the office. These systems wouldn't actually be watching you. They would simply be collecting data behind the scenes in real time to identify disturbances in function—from the expression of your genes to the patterns of your movement. If the system detected a problem, it could notify a family member or community healthcare provider who could reach out to you in person. If the problem required medical attention, you could be seen by a primary care provider in a timely fashion.

We are a little ways out from preventing all chronic disease with early detection and mitigation. As I mentioned, it's just not possible to control all environmental stressors on the human body. So what do we do when a patient actually develops a chronic disease despite our best efforts? We help them *manage* their disease with medications.

But even that's not easy. As we talked about in Chapter 3, I really don't know if any particular medicine is actually going to help an individual patient. In order to best manage chronic disease, we need to know exactly which medicine is going to benefit which patient under which conditions. And that is the very domain of Precision Medicine.

PRECISION MEDICINE AND DISEASE MANAGEMENT

I introduced the concept of precision medicine in Chapter 5, but let's briefly explore how it fits into a reinvented primary care model. Precision, or personalized, medicine refers to how individual patient data—such as genomic or metabolomic data—can be used to customize treatments for individual patients.[151] While precision medicine could apply to any intervention, I will focus on its application in prescribing medications. Let's look at a couple examples of how precision medicine is being used today.

One of the best known applications of precision medicine is drug metabolism. It is well known that patients vary significantly in their response to certain drugs, often because of variants in the gene responsible for metabolizing those drugs. Sometimes, an effective dose for one patient can lead to serious side effects in another. Monitoring drug levels can help, but not all drugs can be monitored easily. By knowing the genetic variants responsible for drug metabolism, specific drugs can be used in specific patients to maximize effectiveness and minimize harm.[152]

Another condition to benefit from precision medicine is cancer. It turns out, it's not just a patient's genome that is unique; a cancer cell has its own unique genome as well. Many different cancers have been studied using precision medicine, including melanoma, colon cancer, lung cancer, and pancreatic cancer. Again, pharmacogenomics could solve the NNT problem; if we knew exactly which chemotherapy agent works for which cancer in which patient, we could avoid prescribing people drugs that will have no effect or, worse, cause harm.[153]

With its focus on individual patients, precision medicine could also transform the way we treat chronic disease and become the foundation of *disease management*. I introduced the term disease management in Chapter 4 when we were talking about on-site health centers. We generally use the term to mean keeping chronic disease "under control." By under control, I mean keeping measures like blood pressure and cholesterol in predefined ranges. But we could also think of disease management as helping a system function most effectively in the setting of unmitigated environmental stressors. Let me share with you how I came to this realization.

One day while I was out rucking, I received a call from a doctor friend of mine at the hospital. I had an older patient hospitalized for *appendicitis*—an infection of the appendix often causing severe abdominal pain. He also had a history of heart disease and kidney disease. My friend was concerned about his rising blood pressure due to all the stress he was under. She wanted to know if I was okay with increasing the dose of his blood pressure medicine to reduce the risk of him having a heart attack or stroke. I told her I thought it was a great idea. I hung up the phone and started thinking as I continued my ruck.

Then it hit me.

This is what I do in my practice every day. I am constantly prescribing medicines to help my patients function as well as possible in the setting of environmental stressors. For example, I prescribe an inhaler for my asthmatic patient who lives in a city with poor air quality to improve their breathing. I prescribe an antidepressant for my patient going through a contentious divorce to improve their mood so they can function at work. I prescribe a diabetes medicine to my patient who cannot reduce their intake of sugar to help their body regulate blood glucose. At the end of the day, I prescribe medications all the time to help my patients cope with environmental stressors they cannot, or choose not to, reduce themselves.

But even this is still a disease-centric model—it focuses on managing individual diseases. Many patients have multiple diseases caused by multiple stressors. How in the world do we handle that? Do we just keep stacking medications one on top of the other for each disease?

Hopefully not for long. Precision medicine and artificial intelligence are evolving, and they stand to dramatically change the way we care for patients. Wearable sensors, including watches and rings, are already available to measure many different physiological systems.[154] And new wearable chemical sensors are being developed that will allow the real-time measurement of biomarkers from many different sources, including blood, sweat, and tears.[155]

I believe that someday we'll be able to integrate all these data sources to develop useful models of individual humans as *whole systems*. These models are often called "medical digital twins," and they could someday improve the treatment of a wide range of medical conditions.[156] They will also allow us to be much more selective in the treatments we recommend to our patients. Perhaps I'll be able to try different interventions on your digital twin to determine the best combination of treatments for your situation, prior to actually trying them on you.

We are a little way out from artificial intelligence advising us on how best to treat our patients, but I believe it will happen. In the meantime, we physicians do have something called *human intelligence*. We are trained to interpret messy data and do our best to apply it to an individual patient sitting in front of us—using both reason *and* intuition.[157] We can talk to patients and identify factors we think are contributing to their conditions. Then we can use our physical exam and lab tests to support or refute our hypotheses. After that, we can develop an individualized plan for our patients using both medical and lifestyle interventions. If something doesn't work, we have new information to make better decisions going forward. This is the *art* side of medicine. It really doesn't require advanced technology, but it does require *time* to understand the context in which a person lives their life.

A primary care model that integrates human intelligence with advances in science, engineering, and technology stands to revolutionize the way we care for patients in this country. Of course, despite our best efforts, patients will still get sick. They will still need procedures and consults from our specialists, or they will get pushed past a tipping point and even need to go to the hospital. When that happens, our role shifts. We go from provider to coordinator.

COORDINATING SPECIALTY CARE

Medical specialists are the experts in our healthcare system. They are physicians and surgeons who receive advanced training—often in one particular organ system of the body. They include such professions as cardiology, gastroenterology, oncology, obstetrics and gynecology, otolaryngology, infectious disease, orthopedics, rheumatology, and so on. Many specialists are affiliated with local community hospitals or academic medical centers. As such, they are sometimes called secondary or tertiary care providers.[158]

As a generalist, I rely on my specialists for problems outside my area of expertise or when my patients need a procedure like a colonoscopy, cardiac catheterization, or surgery. Having a network of medical specialists is critical if I want to provide effective care to my patients. A mentor early in my medical training once told me, "Bill, as a primary care doctor, you are only as good as the specialists around you." There is truth to that. My specialists have bailed me out on many occasions over the years, and I am grateful for all they have done to help me and my patients.

But it works both ways. I need to help my specialists help my patients. This means I *coordinate care* with my specialists, not blindly refer patients to them. This is very different from what we talked about in Chapter 2—punting my patients to specialists because I don't have time to talk with them.

There are a number of ways I try to help my specialists in my current practice. First, I try to make an appropriate referral. It doesn't do anyone any good if I send a patient with a shoulder problem to a surgeon who specializes in knee problems. Second, I try to make sure my specialist has the information they need to do their job—usually a summary of the problem that needs to be addressed and a basic set of tests. Theoretically, this should be taken care of by an electronic medical record system, but if a patient requires an opinion from a specialist in a different health system, they often can't access the records. Third, I follow up on my specialists' recommendations and help with long-term management, such as managing medications. Finally, I try to communicate in an efficient manner. Usually, it's a few quick text messages here and there; occasionally, a short phone conversation.

Make no mistake about it, good communication is critical. I can't count the number of times I have been able to keep a patient out of the hospital by having good communication with my specialists.

The same thing goes for hospital care. When I have a patient who needs to be in the hospital, I want them there—and I am happy to do whatever I can to assist. Usually this means talking with the providers in charge. But as we discussed in Chapter 2, this is often a challenge. It's not much easier after hospitalization either. Coordinating skilled nursing and rehabilitation services either in a facility or at home is no small feat. Still, integrating and coordinating *pre-hospital, hospital, and post-hospital care* is far from impossible. It just requires being advocates for our patients.

As primary care doctors, we should be advocates for our patients. And there is no greater need for this than at the end of one's life. Patient wishes should be honored to the greatest extent possible. Sometimes it's non-negotiable.

A DYING MAN'S WISH

Frank was a seventy-eight-year-old, hard-working, blue-collar guy. When he came to see me, he shared a laundry list of medical conditions he had developed over the years. But it was clear Frank wasn't going to let sickness get in the way of working.

Among other things, Frank had a series of surgeries requiring many blood transfusions, which led to him contracting *hepatitis C*—a chronic viral infection of the liver. This led to *cirrhosis*—impaired liver function due to scar tissue. Unfortunately, Frank wasn't eligible for a liver transplant and his liver disease progressed.

I was with Frank throughout the progression of his liver disease. He was in and out of the hospital several times. During his last hospitalization, things started to progress more quickly: his belly was filling up with fluid, his blood pressure was dropping, his kidney function was declining, his ammonia levels were rising, and he was getting delirious. We were trying to do everything we could, but we got to a point where we knew we weren't going to be able to save him. We had to start thinking about hospice care.

"Dr. Queale, I'm okay with dying," Frank said. "I just want to die at home."

I understood. Frank had a nice little home in the city that was his pride and joy, and I didn't blame him for wanting to go back there. "No problem, Frank. I totally get it. I'll make sure when we get to that point that you're transferred home."

Not too long after, things went downhill fast. As his liver and kidney function ceased and his ammonia levels climbed higher, Frank became unresponsive. I talked to his wife and some other family members, and we made the decision to line up hospice care and get him home.

We got hospice care set up without a problem; all we needed to do was transport him to his home. But we were too late.

Frank was in such poor condition that the hospital discharge planner wouldn't discharge him.

"I'm sorry," she said. "He's not stable enough to transport. We can't send him home. We are going to have to arrange hospice here in the hospital."

"But I promised him that he'd be able to die at home," I told her. She said she was sorry but it was hospital policy. He couldn't go.

His family was there, and they also wanted him to go home. Things started to get a little contentious, so I decided it was best to take the conversation outside of the room. I didn't want Frank to hear this argument, even if he was unconscious.

In the hallway, I said to the nurse, "Listen, I get hospital policy. I really do. But I made this guy a promise. I told him he would be able to die at home. I'll take responsibility if he dies on the way home. I'll even sign a waiver if I have to."

I could tell by the look on her face that she knew I was serious. She told me to hold on and stepped away. She came back five minutes later.

"Okay, you're good to go. I just need you to sign this paperwork. But you have to go now."

Relieved, I went back to the room. Frank was still unresponsive, but I did what I always do in these situations, whether he could hear me or not. Standing by his side, I put my hand on his shoulder and said, "Hey, Frank. It's Bill Queale. Listen, I have some good news for you. You're going home today."

It turned out Frank did hear everything that was going on. To my surprise, he slowly turned his head toward me and opened his eyes ever so slightly. He didn't have the strength to speak, but he mouthed the words.

Thank you.

Frank made it home and died peacefully the following day. Fortunately, I got to see him one more time before he died.

Advocating for patients isn't always easy. And it's nothing we get paid for. But the rewards of successfully fighting on behalf of our patients make it worth the effort.

A SYSTEM-OF-SYSTEMS

Having a strong primary care system as the foundation of a larger American healthcare system just makes sense. And I'm not the only one to think this way. The National Academies of Sciences, Engineering, and Medicine recently addressed this in their 2021 report *Implementing High-Quality Primary Care: Rebuilding the Foundation of Health Care.*[159] This report addressed many of these issues in great detail—defining high-quality primary care; person-centered, family-centered, and community-centered care; integrated primary care delivery; primary care teams; digital health; and something we'll talk about in the next chapter, paying for primary care.

But this still begs the question: *How would we integrate a new primary care model into our broader medical system? What would such a system even look like?*

The answer to that question would come, as it so often does, from one of my kids.

CHAPTER 10

Rebuilding Our Healthcare System

MY YOUNGEST DAUGHTER, ALLY, GRADUATED FROM COL-
lege as a music education major—the furthest thing from being
a doctor! Having no formal music training myself, I learned
a lot during her four years in college. Ally is a clarinetist, and
during her junior year, she was chosen as concertmaster—the
right-hand musician to the conductor.

While I did my best to understand all the technical aspects
of music, I never really understood all the details. But not
knowing the details did not keep me from developing a deep
appreciation for the beautiful sound of a well-conducted symphony orchestra. A symphony orchestra is an incredible display
of individual talent and group cohesion, which together create
an experience with deep beauty, emotion, and meaning.

During one of Ally's performances, I watched her conductor
with amazement. He was incredibly dynamic, moving about

the small podium in synchrony with the music. He was a performance in and of himself. I could see him draw different music sections in and out with specific purpose, occasionally singling out musicians as if to showcase them among the group. While each musician played their individual instrument, they all had their eyes on him as he pulled everyone together to tell a beautiful story.

Then it hit me: *our healthcare system is like a symphony orchestra without a conductor!*

The music is there, and all the musicians are working hard to master their individual parts. But that's the thing—they are only responsible for *their* part. They are only given the notes that *they* need to perform. This is where the conductor comes into play. Someone has to be responsible for pulling all the parts together in perfect timing to produce beautiful music— someone who stands in the center and balances each part of the orchestra. Without a conductor, the cohesion amongst each section is lost.

While a symphony orchestra has strings, trumpets, clarinets, and so on, our healthcare system has cardiologists, gastroenterologists, nephrologists, and so on. And just like the clarinets can't always hear what the trumpets are playing, my cardiology colleagues can't always hear what my nephrology colleagues are saying.

Much like a conductor needs to know something about every instrument, a primary care doctor needs to know something about every specialty. It is my job as a primary care doctor to pull everyone's specialties together, communicating pertinent information in the same way a conductor communicates information to each of their sections. Primary care doctors and conductors serve as hubs in a network through which all information flows and gets redirected in a coordinated fashion.

So can we help our healthcare system produce a beautiful symphony rather than a harsh cacophony? Can we bring order out of disorder? Systems medicine says we can.

The beauty of disorder is that it can lead to reorganization and *regrowth*. But that requires letting go of the past and moving forward in a new direction. And that can provoke fear of the unknown. Still, as they say, *the right thing to do is never the easy thing to do.* Sometimes we just need to get out of our comfort zone.

TAKING ON RISK

In Chapter 4, we talked about *How We Got Here*—how the medical industry evolved and how it has tried to control costs over the years. Let's briefly review what we discussed so that we can better understand how things are changing going forward.

In the early days, medicine was pretty simple. You got sick, you went to a doctor, and somehow you paid for it. As science expanded and the chronic disease epidemic exploded, things got complicated. More sickness created a need for more sick-care services. This led to the discovery of drugs and procedures that cured many diseases, as well as led to the expansion of hospitals and large health systems to provide these services. Next thing you know, we have a multitrillion dollar sickcare system.

But who pays for all these services? *Third party payers*—private insurance companies, Medicare and Medicaid, self-insured corporations, and so on. After collecting money *from you* in the form of taxes or premiums, they pay for medical services delivered *to you* when you need them. If they collect more money in premiums than they spend in medical claims, they make a profit. If not, they go bankrupt. In other words, third party payers are the ones who assume *financial risk* in our healthcare industry.

But managing financial risk is complicated. It's not easy to predict how much money someone is going to spend in any given year. Worse, I don't think anyone a hundred years ago saw the epidemic of chronic disease coming.

As medical costs increased over the past century, insurance companies increased premiums to keep up. More than that, they created all kinds of games to manage risk—HMOs, PPOs, case management, disease management, the Coding Game, copays, high deductibles, you name it. Of course the most notable tactic was reducing the amount of money doctors and hospitals were paid for their services. This forced doctors and hospitals to see more patients to make ends meet. In turn, people only got sicker and medical costs only rose higher. It's been a vicious cycle of increased costs and declining health for the past fifty years.

But the tide is changing.

Value-based care is encouraging the shift of financial risk from payers to providers in exchange for potential rewards. As we discussed, the most well-known example of this is the Accountable Care Organization (ACO). But while ACOs seem to provide better care at a lower cost, they have not fundamentally changed the game. They have, however, given us insight into the solution to our problem.

And what we have learned is this: *when you incentivize a group of medical providers to provide high-value care, they figure out how to provide high-value care.*

So, if transferring risk (and reward) to providers is working, why not go further? Why not share *more* of the money collected in premiums and taxes and let *them* help manage the financial risk. Well, this is actually what is starting to happen. These are often called *capitated models* and they are getting some attention.[160] Medicare's ACO REACH program and Medicare Advantage Plans have already started shifting risk to providers, and commercial plans are following.[161]

Of course, all this does is shift more financial risk to providers. By itself, it doesn't reduce the risk. Furthermore, medical providers—such as large regional health systems—are not used to managing that kind of financial risk. In fact, the whole idea of being on the hook for all medical expenses in a population is downright scary.

While we often talk about *upside risk*—the opportunity to make money by providing high-quality care—large provider groups worry about *downside risk*, the possibility they could lose money if they don't provide good care, or simply have a string of bad luck. So how can providers minimize the downside risk associated with total medical costs? One way is to have specialized insurance policies to cover these worst-case scenarios. But there is another way:

They could invest in a new primary care model.

The best way to reduce the downside risk of paying for all medical costs in a population is to end the epidemic of chronic disease that drives up costs in the first place. And this is the jurisdiction of primary care. Primary care providers need to partner with payers and share in the financial risk of paying for total medical costs of a population. Then they can partner with hospitals, specialists, technology companies, and allied health professionals to form various types of *Risk-Bearing Entities (RBEs)*—networks of organizations that all assume financial risk for the total cost of medical care in a population.[162]

New value-based care arrangements with a focus on primary care seem to be the direction things are headed. The Centers for Medicare and Medicaid (CMS) Innovation Center recently published its strategy for achieving equitable outcomes through high-quality, affordable, person-centered care.[163] The goal is to have all Medicare and Medicaid beneficiaries in value-based care by 2030.

Another group to jump on the bandwagon is *private equity*— financial firms that pool money together from investors, then invest the money in businesses to make a profit. Healthcare, after all, is a business, and it appears primary care is the next big investment opportunity. US companies focused on primary care raised about $16 billion from investors in 2021 alone.[164] But we should be extremely careful here. Private equity is a double-edged sword. While the right private-equity partner with the right mission could help reduce inefficiencies and spur innovation, the wrong partner could focus more on short-term profits rather than long-term, high-quality patient care.[165]

By managing the flow of money within their network of providers, RBEs could decide how best to allocate funds to maximize efficiencies in the delivery of care to their population of patients. After all, every community is different and has its own unique needs and resources at various points in time. Such a decentralized approach to healthcare delivery could make health systems more adaptable to changes in local conditions, in turn making them more resilient. Now that's a systems approach to healthcare delivery.

Of course, since RBEs are in charge of paying themselves for the care they provide to patients, they will need to ask themselves the question, *How much money should we spend on primary care anyway?* Let's take a look at some options.

PAYING FOR PRIMARY CARE

Right now, on average, primary care consumes around 5–7 percent of all healthcare dollars spent in this country.[166] That's roughly $200–$300 billion. Studies show it should probably be twice that much if we really want to make an impact.[167]

If I am advising a regional health system on how much to spend on primary care, I am using these numbers. Whatever is being spent currently, *double it.* The state of Rhode Island did this as part of their Care Transformation Collaborative and realized a 250 percent return on their investment.[168]

The extra investment in primary care could be used to finance a reinvented primary care model that would

- expand a workforce of office- and community-based primary care providers;
- increase the salaries of primary care physicians to those comparable to their specialists;
- invest in an expanded primary care team, including nurse practitioners and physician assistants, registered nurses, social workers, behavioral health specialists, dietitians, physical therapists, and pharmacists;
- develop programs that promote a healthy lifestyle as much as prescribing medications;
- expand a team of administrative personnel who manage primary care practices and help coordinate care for complex patients; and
- invest in technology to develop disease prevention, early detection, and mitigation algorithms, as well as to help scale services to all members of a community.

Only by investing in a new primary care model will investors see a significant return on their investment in a healthcare system that takes on financial risk.

This all sounds very nice, but RBEs will still have to address the specific question, *How do we actually compensate primary care providers for the work they do?* Clearly, fee-for-service doesn't work. There are a number of opinions out there, but here are my suggestions:

First, pay primary care practices a fixed monthly fee for each patient under their care. This covers practice overhead, advanced technology, an expanded team of providers, and the multitude of administrative tasks performed on a daily basis—tasks that could never be assigned a billing code. These *capitated payments* allow providers to see fewer patients per day and spend more time with each patient. They also guarantee some level of practice income that is not dependent on patient volume. Capitated payments saved many practices during the pandemic when patients were not going to see their doctors.[169] Some suggest capitated payments should be risk-adjusted, but this gets complicated. There are other ways to help adjust for patient complexity, which leads me to my next point.

Second, pay providers on a fee-for-service basis for time they spend with their patients. But wait, *I thought fee-for-service was bad!* By itself, it's bad, but at the same time, primary care providers need to be paid for the work they do. Let's face it, some patients are challenging and require a significant amount of time to stabilize, heal, and rebuild their lives. If a provider is not going to get paid more for doing more work, many just won't do the work. We can talk about ethics all day long, but it's just human nature. Plus, a fee-for-service helps solve the risk adjustment issue. The more time a provider spends with a patient managing a complex condition, the more they get paid.

Finally, offer a bonus payment to *all providers* in a Risk-Bearing Entity—primary care, specialists, hospital, and allied health providers—based on the savings generated by providing high-quality care to the whole population. This will encourage everyone to *cooperate* with each other to keep people healthy and out of the hospital. And unlike the old HMO days, it incentivizes providers to do the right thing for their patients, not restrict care in order to save money. In other words, if I think an MRI, a pacemaker, or hospitalization is the right thing to do for my patient, I am going to do it. If not, I won't.

There is something else to consider here. Perhaps patients should be part of this financial model, too. Maybe they should receive a rebate on their insurance premium at the end of the year if they actively participate in their care—engaging with their primary care providers, living a healthy lifestyle, taking their medications, and keeping appointments with their specialists. Maybe for the first time ever, insurance premiums could go *down* instead of up over the years.

As healthcare dollars move away from fee-for-service toward value-based arrangements, we have an opportunity to build a new primary care system that serves as the foundation of a larger coordinated medical system—a system that focuses on *healthcare* as much as it does *sickcare*. Perhaps with such a coordinated system in place, we could finally end the epidemic of chronic disease and reduce the suffering of so many people in this country.

Of course, creating such a coordinated system is not without its challenges. It couldn't be that easy, could it? Let's quickly run through a few of these challenges and see if we can solve them ahead of time.

ROADBLOCKS TO IMPLEMENTATION

No solution comes problem-free. If we're successful in scaling a new coordinated healthcare system, we create at least three problems. First, if each provider sees fewer patients per day, we'll need more primary care providers. Second, we will need to train primary care providers in a new systems-based delivery of care. Third, we'll need to figure out what to do with all the empty hospital beds and extra staff as we reduce the number of avoidable hospitalizations. Let's take a look at these one at a time.

I've argued time and time again that the problem with our current primary care system is one of high volume. However, if we reduce the number of patients a primary care doctor sees in any given day, it stands to reason that we will need more primary care doctors. And since we are already slated to have a shortage of between 21,400 and 55,200 primary care physicians by 2033, it looks like we could be compounding the problem.[170]

There are a few ways we can solve this problem. First, we can and should use nurse practitioners and physician assistants to help doctors see patients in the office setting. This is not pushing high volume onto our medical colleagues; it is dividing the same number of patients by more providers. Second, as we discussed, a reinvented primary care system could include an entirely new workforce of community-based providers. This workforce could serve as an extension of the primary care team and work with patients and families in their own homes and communities. Establishing such a workforce could also solve an economic problem by providing entry-level jobs for people who want to get into healthcare as a career but might not otherwise have the opportunity. Finally, as automated primary care platforms come to fruition, the number of patients seen by a primary care *system* could be substantial. With a team of office-based, community-based, and technology-based providers, all members of a community could have access to a primary care *system* under the supervision of one primary care physician.

There is one other source of primary care doctors I should mention—specialists. Many doctors choose medical specialties like cardiology and gastroenterology simply because they can make more money than they can in primary care. I can assure you, if doctors can make more money practicing primary care than specialty care, you'll very quickly have more primary care doctors.

The second problem we face with rebuilding our healthcare system is that we have an entire workforce of primary care providers trained in a conventional model of care—a model heavily focused on prescribing drugs based on population health guidelines. As we move toward technology-enabled care of individual patients, including precision medicine treatments and lifestyle interventions, providers will need to be re-educated. In the short term, I suspect continuing education courses will emerge focusing more specifically on systems medicine, systems biology, precision medicine, lifestyle medicine, and community health. Long term, however, we will need systems thinking to be formally integrated into our medical school curricula.

Fortunately, as we talked about in Chapter 5, efforts are already underway through the *American Medical Association (AMA) Accelerating Change in Medical Education Initiative.*[171] This initiative is working across a continuum of partners to bring health systems science into the medical school curricula. The hope is that by doing so, physicians and other health professionals will be able to deliver higher-value care to their patients and communities. I suspect they will.

This brings us to the third problem. By radically reducing the number of sick people that currently depend on our sickcare system, we run the risk of crippling our current hospital-based healthcare industry. While I would anticipate a reduction in avoidable hospitalizations and potential downsizing of hospitals, I don't believe the implementation of a new primary care model will mark the end of the hospital industry. Instead, I believe it would be the beginning of a new and vastly improved hospital industry.

Right now, hospitals are basically *high-volume, low-margin businesses*—meaning they see a lot of patients and don't make a large profit margin.[172] And, as we have seen, hospitals are filled with patients who don't need to be there. Under new financial models, hospitals could become *low-volume, high-margin businesses*—meaning they will see fewer patients but make higher profits by providing more advanced services. In other words, although the cost of hospital care might increase per patient, it would be offset by the reduced patient volume and increased value it provides to patients overall. Plus, since hospitals would be partners in new risk-bearing entities, they would benefit financially by supporting their primary care providers in the outpatient setting. *In effect, hospitals could make more money by keeping people out of the hospital!*

There will likely be hospital closures, though. Buildings will go vacant, and staff will be laid off. But there will be plenty of opportunities to repurpose hospital buildings in ways that could improve their local communities. Maybe we could use them for homeless shelters or drug treatment centers; we could surely use more of them. As for any staff layoffs that might occur, there will be no shortage of new jobs for healthcare workers; I predict more primary care services will be offered in the home and community, creating demand for a new workforce of community-based healthcare providers.

Arguably the greatest roadblock to change is change itself. As bad as a situation might be, it always seems easier to go along with the status quo. But if we can create a healthcare system that allows people to make more money keeping people *healthy* than treating them after they get *sick*, I can assure you the system will change.

Actually, the system already appears to be changing. Evidence is coming in that high-quality primary care improves access, provides better care coordination, and lowers costs.[173] But I don't need numbers to tell me the model works. I knew it sixteen years ago after receiving a phone call that would change the entire way I thought about this problem.

THE MODEL WORKS

In Chapter 3, I told you how I was nearly bankrupted by insurance companies and almost quit medicine altogether. Instead, I decided to start over and create a new medical practice model focused on providing high quality of care to a smaller group of patients.

Two years into my new model, I got a call from the credentialing coordinator at one of my local hospitals. Her job was to renew my hospital privileges.

"Hey Bill, you're up for renewal of your privileges," she said. "I'm doing the paperwork, and I just need to know how many patients you've admitted to our hospital over the past year."

I thought about it for a moment and then told her I didn't think I had admitted anybody.

"Nobody?" she said in disbelief.

"Nobody," I repeated.

"That's a problem," she said bluntly.

"How could that be a problem?"

"I can't renew your hospital privileges if you don't admit any patients to the hospital."

"With all due respect, what do you want me to do? Make people sick just so that I can admit them and get privileges?"

We both laughed at such a ridiculous notion. But we had a real problem and she wasn't sure what to do. I didn't want to lose my hospital privileges; I had a great network of specialists to work with, and I used the hospital often for labs, MRIs, and other procedures. I was giving them plenty of business, and they were providing great services to my patients. It was a great partnership. We had to figure this one out.

"Well, how about other admissions?" she said. "Do you have patients admitted for other services?"

"Sure," I said. "I often refer patients to my surgical colleagues who perform elective procedures like total joint replacements, hernia repairs, or gallbladder resections."

She asked if I ever visited my patients in the hospital. I told her I did, all the time.

"There we go, then! Next time you admit someone to another doctor's service, even though you're not the attending physician, just go in and write a note in the chart. This will show the hospital that you're actually sending patients there and that the hospital is making money." The problem was solved.

The fact that I hadn't admitted any patients to my service at my local hospital for a year suggested I was on to something. Everything I discussed in the past two chapters—creating a relationship with my patients, preventing disease or catching it early, treating diseases with medications *and* lifestyle interventions, and coordinating care with my specialists—could keep patients healthy and out of the hospital altogether.

I knew in my heart—*the model works.*

A FEW MORE THOUGHTS

The healthcare conundrum we discussed in Part I of this book is not insurmountable. I believe the combination of *systems thinking* and *value-based care* could rebuild our healthcare system from the bottom up. In other words, with the right policies and incentives in place, the problem basically takes care of itself.

But while writing this book, it occurred to me that if we truly want to rebuild our healthcare system, we have some decisions to make at multiple levels—as individuals, a healthcare system, and society as a whole. After all, the words in this book are useless if we don't act on them.

My conclusion takes a slight twist. I would like to explore the choices we have in front of us at multiple levels and how they might all be connected. And I'd like to start with a story about a struggling patient of mine named Mike.

Conclusion

THE CHOICE

MIKE WAS A HEALTHY MAN IN HIS LATE THIRTIES. HE WAS married with three children and had a high-stress job in cybersecurity. When he first came to see me, I could tell right away he really didn't want to be there. Many men just don't like to go to the doctor—me included! But Mike and I hit it off. I focused my attention on common interests and built the relationship from there.

Over the years, I noticed Mike getting more withdrawn. He wouldn't look me in the eye as much, and he would skirt conversation. Because of his change in behavior, I wondered if alcohol was playing a role. But he denied it was a problem, so I didn't press it; after all, it was just a hunch.

Soon Mike's health started to decline. He was hospitalized three times for *pancreatitis*—a condition often caused by drinking too much alcohol. Then he started having trouble in his marriage. All the while, he continued to deny alcohol was a problem. Then one day, I got a call that Mike crashed his car while driving drunk. Now he was facing charges of driving while intoxicated.

I was able to convince Mike to go to rehab and helped coordinate an admission to the same treatment center I had attended twenty years earlier. Mike gave me permission to talk with his counselor so that I could be involved in his care.

A week into his stay, Mike's counselor told me things weren't going very well. While Mike was cordial and respectful, he wasn't very engaged. Then, I was told that he wanted to leave. Honestly, I took it a bit personally, given the work I had done to get him in there. So I decided to pay Mike a visit to see what was going on.

When I got there, the counselor told me that Mike did not see the value of the lectures and meetings he was required to attend. She asked me to sit in a little white room while she went to get Mike and bring him in. Mike didn't know I was coming, so you can imagine the surprise on his face when he walked into the room and saw me sitting there. He looked terrible. He had a hoodie on and was all slumped over. His eyes were sunken, and he looked tired.

"How's it going?" I asked him.

"Not great," he responded. "This place is a waste of my time. I have nothing to learn from those people out there."

That comment hit me hard. Not only had I spent three years

working with an incredible leadership team to provide good care to our patients, I was one of "those people" myself years earlier. But in all honesty, I understood how he felt. When I went to rehab, I too didn't think I had much to learn. Sure, I was glad to be removed from society and put into a protected environment with other struggling people—but *learn* something from them? I was a doctor, for God's sake. What was I going to learn from a bunch of drug addicts?

My mind went rapidly back and forth, between anger at Mike for disrespecting a place I loved and compassion for another struggling addict. The thought occurred to me that maybe I should tell him that I had once been a patient there and that I knew how he felt. But that would require coming clean to one of my patients. If word got out that I was a recovering drug addict, my reputation could be seriously damaged.

All of this went through my mind in a matter of seconds. I felt a sense of panic. I didn't know how to respond.

"Yeah, that's how I felt when I was here," I said, surprising myself that I even said it.

"Wait, you went here?" he asked me in disbelief.

"Yeah, about twenty years ago. And 'those people' you talk about out there? They saved my life. And they are some of my best friends to this day." I paused. "Listen, I'm not going to tell you what to do. You can leave here anytime you want. But you might want to stay and see if there is something you can learn from 'those people' out there. You might be surprised."

I started walking to the door but turned back to add one more thing: "Oh and by the way, if you do decide to leave, you can be assured your wife and kids won't stick around. They won't put up with your bullshit anymore. It's your choice, but I suggest you give it a shot."

Mike didn't say anything after that. I wished him good luck and left the room.

Mike did, in fact, choose to stay in rehab. Not only that, he embraced a program of recovery as well as anyone I had ever met. Mike *made changes to the way he lived his life,* and he is now on a path of healing from his addiction to alcohol.

Did my decision to confess my past have anything to do with his decision to stay? I don't really know. But it had a positive effect on me. Confessing my story to a patient released a secret I had been keeping from the public for twenty years. They say, *you are only as sick as your secrets.* Well, I took a chance that day. I exposed a secret and took another step forward on my own path of healing.

We all have decisions to make about our health. We can continue living our lives as we are, taking more and more drugs when we get sick—or we can make changes to the way we live our lives and heal from our chronic dis-ease.

We have decisions to make as a healthcare system as well. We can stay wedded to our fee-for service financial models and profit off people being sick—or we can embrace value-based financial models and profit from people being healthy.

But those are not the only choices we have in front of us. Let's be honest—we are not doing so well as a species. The world is changing rapidly, and we seem to be getting more and more stressed. It might even be changing faster than we can adapt.[174] If that's the case, who knows what could happen next?

OUR ENVIRONMENT IS CHANGING

As I have discussed throughout this book, chronic disease and chronic dis-ease are often the result of excessive environmental stressors in genetically susceptible people. I really don't need fancy science or technology to tell me this. I see it every day in my practice.

In talking with my patients recently, it seems that environmental stressors are *increasing* in our society, not decreasing. For one thing, our climate really is changing. While people can argue all day long about *why* it's changing, it is changing.[175] There certainly could be more and worse storms, droughts, extreme heat, and extreme flooding on the horizon. We also live in a world of emerging viruses, and we're likely to have more pandemics. I hate to say it, but COVID-19 is nothing compared to what could be lurking around the corner. In addition, we'll be producing more chemicals and plastics that will further stress our systems. And social media is only going to push us further to the political extremes.

You don't have to be a social science expert to know that there's a lot of dis-ease out there. All you have to do is turn on the news or scroll through social media. Everybody is resorting to their tribe and falling prey to confirmation bias. Everything seems to be a debate between two groups who are diametrically opposed but believe they are 100 percent correct.

You can't have a conversation with someone if you outright dismiss everything they think and believe. You can't form friendships, forge policy, or even just have a friendly chat with someone over a cup of coffee. *Is there any middle ground anymore?*

Unchecked, all these stressors are only going to challenge our health further—physically, mentally, and socially.[176] If we don't change course soon, these increasing stressors could push us *all* closer to a tipping point.

In fact, it's so bad that some people think we need to colonize another planet to carry on our human legacy.[177] I have more faith in us than that. I think we can turn things around. A coordinated healthcare system built on a foundation of primary care could certainly help.

But there are plenty of legitimate reasons to send humans into space.[178] For one thing, many of the challenges with providing medical care in space are similar to those we face here on Earth—such as preventing acute injuries and illness requiring hospitalization. This presents an opportunity for scientists, engineers, and physicians to work together to solve problems in both areas. But regardless of any technical reason, we humans are just driven to explore, and space is the next frontier.

A HEALTHCARE SYSTEM IN SPACE

While I may never have realized my dream of being an astronaut,

I have recently had the privilege of working with many experts involved in human spaceflight. It turns out space is an extremely high-stress environment. With little or no gravity, high levels of radiation, a lack of air, and severely cold temperatures, surviving outside Earth's atmosphere is not easy. We could choose to stay here where it is comfortable—but we are going.

It's one thing to send a spacecraft into space, but sending *humans* into space is a whole other ballgame. It's hard to overstate how dangerous and improbable it is to do such a feat successfully. There are the environmental stressors mentioned above, but there are also other factors to contend with. We humans are kind of dirty—with our trillions of bacteria, viruses, and parasites that we carry as part of our microbiome. And even the most well-trained astronauts need to eat, sleep, and use a bathroom. Plus, we humans get tired, cranky, and lonely. We also get sick and injured.

However, none of that is going to stop us. The Artemis program is already underway and we are headed back to the Moon for sure. In fact, there are already plans to build a permanent lunar base station.[179] But even the Moon is only three days away. In case of an emergency, we could design a medical spacecraft to get astronauts back to Earth if needed—a space ambulance of sorts.

A crew traveling to Mars, however, is on their own. Sure, there would be some medical supplies onboard, but not many. And there's no turning around quickly to come home. Add to that a delay in communication of up to twenty minutes—forty minutes round trip—and there is no physician immediately available to help in an emergency.[180]

This creates a challenge. *How do we mitigate the risk of a serious medical event that jeopardizes the health of the crew and success of the mission?*

Since we know environmental stressors account for most injuries and illnesses, I suspect the spacecraft environment and crew lifestyle will be important—including spacecraft design, daily work routines, regular exercise, proper nutrition, adequate sleep, and positive relationships with other crew members. While astronauts will need to operate at peak performance, they will also need to minimize environmental stressors to minimize the risk of disease. In other words, we can't just create a reactive medical system in space. We need astronauts to never get sick in the first place.

One solution might look something like the *Smart Medical Home* we discussed in Chapter 9. For an extended period of time, astronauts would work and live together in a contained environment, much in the way patients and families live in their own home. As a result, astronauts would have to care for each other in their own living space—but they would need some kind of automated primary care system to help them. They would need advanced sensors to monitor crew activity and identify when someone is approaching a critical threshold—or tipping point. Then they would need computer algorithms to analyze all the potential contributing factors that caused the disturbance and assign a treatment plan to restore homeostasis with the highest probability of success. And all this would need to be individualized to each astronaut.

Sadly, we would also need a compassionate hospice process. Some astronauts will likely die in deep space—especially in early Mars missions. We have to make sure they don't suffer and that remaining crew members can heal and move on with their mission.

By working together, I believe scientists, engineers, and physicians can solve the challenges of human spaceflight. I have no doubt we will successfully send humans to Mars (and get them back) in my lifetime.

But we shouldn't have to leave planet Earth to create a healthy civilization. Frankly, if we don't figure it out here, we are only going to re-create a dysfunctional society somewhere else. Just ask any addict who has traveled from city to city looking for things to get better, only to keep repeating the same behaviors that caused their problems in the first place. If we really want peace on Earth, or any other planet for that matter, it has to start from within.

A NEW FOUNDATION

When I was in the thick of my active addiction, I engaged in some pretty unhealthy behaviors. And for those I hurt during that time I am deeply, deeply sorry. The fact is, like most addicts, I needed to make some changes.

But change is hard. *We resist!* We hold onto behaviors that give us pleasure or relieve us of pain! The problem is, we keep aging and our environment keeps changing around us. Over time, behaviors that might have worked well in a previous environment don't work very well in our current environment. In fact, sometimes they work against us.

Of course, it doesn't need to be this way. At any point in

time, we can change the trajectory of our lives. Sometimes that requires medications, hospitalizations, or surgery. Other times it requires taking inventory of our own behaviors and our relationships with people around us. The fact is, sometimes we need to let unhealthy behaviors and relationships die before we can create new ones and move forward with a new life. This metaphorical process of dying means we *simplify* our lives by *detaching* from stressors that caused our dysfunction in the first place. Once our stressors are reduced, we can heal and move forward in a new direction.

This also suggests that chronic dis-ease has a purpose. It tells us that what we are doing is not working. We need to change. And we *can* change. Whether you choose science or faith to explain it, pain and suffering really can be transformed into meaning and purpose.

Of course helping navigate this process is what we want to do for our patients. *This is the essence of primary care!* But our primary care system is broken. It's not working. Primary care itself needs to change. We need to reinvent the primary care model and return it to its natural place as the primary point of contact with our medical system—the interface between 330 million Americans and a multitrillion dollar sickcare system. Every person in this country should have access to a primary care *system* that can see them as a whole and unique person and help improve their health with medical *and* lifestyle interventions.

Since society is a network of people, maybe we could all benefit by being healthier. If we were healthier as individuals, maybe our interactions with one another would be more constructive. Maybe we would find some forgiveness for one another, instead of tearing each other apart so much. Maybe we could work together to solve the problems we are about to face as a planet, or at least help each other adapt to a changing global environment. Because I can assure you, change is coming.

Whether it is us as individuals, the American healthcare system, or society as a whole, we are all complex systems subjected to changing environmental conditions. And we all have a choice. We can either adapt to new conditions by making changes to the way we live our lives, or we can forge ahead with the status quo, blaming everyone else for our problems. If we do the latter, the house of cards will fall someday. And only God knows what that looks like.

But even then, if we survive, we'll be okay. Like the flat sand at low tide, we'll have a new foundation upon which to rebuild. The only question then will be, *what do we build on our new foundation?*

Glossary

Accountable Care Organization, or ACO: A value-based care model in which providers and payers are incentivized to work together and share data to deliver better care to their patients.

Activities of Daily Living, or ADLs: The set of activities we all engage in on a daily basis.

Advanced ADLs: Activities that are important to a person—the essence of a meaningful life—such as gardening, dancing, hiking, camping, volunteer work, traveling, recreational sports, or just playing with grandchildren.

Appendicitis: An infection of the appendix often causing severe abdominal pain.

Aspiration Pneumonia: A condition where fluid enters the trachea or windpipe, causing inflammation or infection in the lungs.

Autoimmune Disease: A condition where the immune system attacks the very body it's supposed to protect.

Automated Care: Primary care services that are offered directly to patients by computer algorithms.

Autophagy: A dynamic recycling process that produces new building blocks and energy for cellular renovation and homeostasis.

Basic ADLs: Activities required for self-care, such as getting in and out of bed, walking short distances, using the bathroom, and eating.

Benefits Consultant: A person who helps companies provide benefits to their employees.

Bowel Obstruction: A blocked intestine.

Brain Aneurysm: A bulge in an artery in the brain.

Cardiac Catheterization: A procedure where they place a catheter into the coronary arteries and look for a blocked artery.

Caste System: A hierarchical system of social and economic status.

Chronic Disease: A persistent condition that limits daily living or requires ongoing medical attention, such as obesity, diabetes, heart disease, cancer, dementia, and arthritis.

Chronic Dis-ease: A general sense of uneasiness and despair that defies any actual diagnosis.

Chronic Stress: Constant pressure that consumes us on a day-to-day basis.

Circadian Rhythms: Our bodies' natural response to the cycle of light and dark.

Cirrhosis: Impaired liver function due to scar tissue.

Community: A network of people that emerges in society based on shared values, beliefs, and interests.

Compression of Morbidity: Minimizing disease and disability to the smallest amount possible and pushing it to the very end of your life.

Confirmation Bias: Believing anything that supports our self-narrative, positive or negative, and dismissing anything that argues against it.

Connections: Links between parts in a network.

Deoxyribonucleic Acid, or DNA: A molecule that contains the genes that code for little proteins called enzymes, which drive chemical reactions.

Disorder: System behavior that is less predictable, haphazard, and sometimes destructive.

Dopamine: A chemical messenger in the brain that manages the delicate balance between pleasure and pain.

Downside Risk: The possibility that providers could lose money if they don't provide good care, or simply have a string of bad luck.

Dynamic: Changes over time.

Early Detection and Mitigation: Detecting disease as early as possible and intervening before it gets out of control.

Environment: Anything outside of a system's distinct boundaries.

Environmental Stressors: Anything that puts stress on biological systems.

Enzymes: Specialized protein molecules that regulate biochemical reactions.

Epidemiology: The study of how diseases are distributed in large populations.

Estimation: The process when researchers put sample data into a mathematical model.

Evidence-Based Medicine: A medical decision-making practice based on formal research.

Fee-for-Service: A method of paying medical providers by assigning a fee for medical services provided to patients.

Frailty: The susceptibility to disease.

Free Radical: A highly unstable molecule that can cause damage to organs in the body.

Functional Training: Dynamic activities performed in a complex environment, often with other people, with a focus on balance, coordination, and agility.

Gatekeepers: Point guards navigating patient care.

Health Information Portability and Accountability Act, or HIPAA: A law designed to protect patient privacy.

Health Maintenance Organization, or HMO: An insurance model in which primary care doctors worked directly for insurance companies to control costs.

Heat Stroke: A potentially lethal condition from being overheated.

Hepatitis C: A chronic viral infection of the liver.

High Intensity Interval Training: Engaging in brief intervals of exercise—such as running, cycling, or rowing—at a faster pace to burn carbohydrates for energy.

Holism: A science that seeks to understand you as a whole person.

Homeostasis: The process of maintaining normal function in a biological system.

Hospital Readmission Rate: A quality measure used to track the number of patient readmissions to hospitals after discharge.

Hospitalist: A physician who specializes in hospital medicine.

Inpatient Hospice: A healthcare facility that specializes in helping people die with peace, comfort, and dignity.

Instrumental ADLs: Activities required for independent living, such as shopping, cooking, dressing, and managing finances.

Intermittent Fasting: Structured periods of time when you are not eating any calories.

Intussusception: A condition where the small intestine "telescopes" inside itself, causing an obstruction or blockage of the bowel.

Irritable Bowel Syndrome, or IBS: A collection of abdominal symptoms that defy a more specific diagnosis.

Lifestyle Intervention: An attempt to restore health through nutrition, exercise, sleep, and improved relationships with other people.

Low Intensity Exercise: Also known as endurance training, exercises that you can perform for a long period of time while carrying on a conversation, such as a brisk walk or riding a stationary bike.

Medicaid Managed Care Organization, or Medicaid MCO:

Private health plans that receive money from the government to take care of Medicaid patients.

Medical Claim: A paper or electronic document that tells an insurance company what service was provided and for what reason.

Medical-Industrial Complex: A system that includes large hospitals, nursing homes, pharmaceutical companies, medical equipment companies, and insurance companies.

Medicare Advantage: A program where Medicare contracts with private insurance companies who pay for medical services to Medicare beneficiaries.

Metabolic Flexibility: The ability to go back and forth between burning carbohydrates and fat for energy.

Microbiome: A massive ecosystem of microorganisms that we carry along with us all the time.

Mitochondria: Power plants inside cells that convert the food we eat into energy to do work.

Mononucleosis: A viral infection common in children and teenagers.

Moral Injury: The result of engaging in or witnessing behaviors that go against an individual's core values or moral beliefs.

Mutation: An abnormality in gene structure.

Network: A set of parts connected together to form a distinct entity.

Nurse Practitioner, or NP: A registered nurse who received advanced training to provide medical services.

Order: System behavior that is somewhat regular and predictable.

Palliative Care Doctor: A physician who specializes in relieving discomfort toward the end of someone's life.

Pancreatitis: A condition often caused by drinking too much alcohol.

Payer: Anyone who is footing the bill for medical expenses, whether an insurance company, government program, private organization, or individual.

Pharmacogenomics: A field that uses genomics to inform drug dosing decisions.

Pharmacology: A field that teaches medical providers how to prescribe medications appropriately.

Post-Traumatic Stress Disorder, or PTSD: A condition that may occur in people who have experienced or witnessed a traumatic event.

Potentially Avoidable Hospitalization: A situation where a patient might have avoided being admitted to a hospital, had they previously received preventative care or treatment.

Precision Medicine: A field that uses personalized data to tailor medical treatments to individual patients or groups of patients.

Preferred Provider Organization, or PPO: An insurance model in which doctors sign a contract agreeing to certain fees for services in exchange for being included in a company's provider network.

Private Equity: A financial firm that pools money together from investors, then invests the money in businesses to make a profit.

Provider: A person or organization that renders healthcare services to patients.

Psychological Stress: Stress that results from navigating the demands of our modern life.

Quality Measures: Numbers referring to a particular area of interest, such as medication errors or hospital infection rates.

Randomized Controlled Trial, or RCT: An advanced study design used to determine if a drug is effective, with minimal bias.

Recovery: The process of changing behaviors and healing from addiction.

Reductionism: The science of breaking things down into smaller and smaller parts to understand how something works at the lowest level.

Resentment: Deep-seated anger for harm that was done to us in the past.

Resilience: The ability to avoid injury or illness under high-stress conditions.

Resistance Training: Pushing, pulling, and lifting against some type of resistance like dumbbells, rubber bands, or just your own body weight.

Risk-Bearing Entity, or RBE: A network of organizations that all assume financial risk for the total cost of medical care in a population.

Sarcopenia: Loss of muscle mass.

Sickcare: A medical system that makes a lot of money off people being sick.

Stress Fracture: Small fractures of a bone, often due to repeated impact with the ground.

Stress Ulcer: Mild bleeding caused by excess stomach acid.

Systems Biology: A scientific field that studies complex biological systems through the interaction of many biomolecules.

Systems Medicine: A field that seeks to understand human health and disease as emergent properties from within.

Third Party Payer: An organization that collects money from people then reimburses a doctor for providing services to them.

Tipping Point: A sudden and dramatic shift in system behavior under increasing amounts of stress.

Trajectory: The course a disease takes over time.

Upside Risk: The opportunity to make money by providing high-quality care.

Value: The amount of positive results per dollar spent.

Acknowledgments

THIS BOOK HAS BEEN A MASSIVE ENDEAVOR, AND I COULD never have pulled it off without the help and support of an incredible number of people.

I have to first thank my good friend Joe Mechlinski, who suggested I write this book. You told me I had to get all this stuff out of my head, and you were right. Thank you for your support, brother.

To my team at Scribe, including Neddie Ann Underwood, Fredric Sinclair, Barbara Boyd, Joy Yeou, Cristina Ricci, Anna Dorfman, Kathleen McIntosh, Jessica Findley, Carla Counsil, Natalia Pagán Serrano, and Zoe Ratches. Your support, advice, and professionalism through this process are incredibly appreciated. I know I haven't been the easiest client, and I am grateful for your patience with me.

To all my content experts and beta readers, including Gary Riccio, Mark Shelhamer, Collan Rosier, Hope Keller, Chris

Bradburne, Hunter Young, Greg Hobelmann, Mark Watson, Bob Cawley, Charlene Frizzera, Marty Makary, Marjorie Rodgers Cheshire, Dan and Sandy Krivit, Dave Gallitano, Corey Hall, Kevin Grodnitzky, Devon Dobrosielski, Erin Prokop, Larry Dukes, Gerry Sandusky, Marjorie Rodgers-Cheshire, and Greg Valcourt. You all gave up your valuable time to help me, and your comments and feedback made this a much better book.

To my friends in recovery who keep me from going off the rails, especially my sponsor Fred H., and my friends Anthony W., Dave D., Jimmy R., Edward W., Bryan S., Pete V., Barry M., Scott T., and Frank S. You guys have been there at some of my darkest times and never gave up on me. You are my brothers, and I love you all.

To all those who have guided me in my spiritual journey, especially Father Mike Schleupner, Father Patrick Carrion, Father Chuck Wible, Father Jack Podsiadlo, and Mr. John Weetenkamp. I am closer to God because of all of you, and I am grateful for our conversations and correspondences over the years.

To all my patients current and past, who have invited me into your lives at some of your most intimate moments. I have learned so much from each and every one of you, and I am grateful for the opportunity to be part of your journey.

To my father, Bill, and my brother, Bob, who both have endured me spouting off time and time again and whose advice on many issues has helped me get through some tough times. Thank you both for always being there for me.

To my mother, Harriett, whose unconditional love I still feel, even though you departed us many years ago. I love you, and I miss you.

To my mother-in-law, Yvonne, who took my mother's place here on Earth. Your love for me is so genuine, and I am grateful.

To my children, Julia, Elliot, Lauren, and Ally. I love each of you more than you will ever know. Thank you for so many amazing memories, and I look forward to many more to come. I am indebted to all of you for your help with my book and patience with me throughout this process.

Finally, and most importantly, to my wife, Karen. No one has suffered more over the past three years while I was writing this book than you. You have had to endure endless hours of me sitting at my desk typing and sighing, or walking around ranting and raving. You are my rock. You are my soulmate. I love you, and I thank you so much for your unwavering support during this journey.

Notes

1   Department of Justice, Drug Enforcement Administration, "Drug Fact Sheet: Stimulants," April 2020, https://www.dea.gov/sites/default/files/2020-06/Stimulants-2020.pdf.

2   "About Chronic Diseases," National Center for Chronic Disease Prevention and Health Promotion, U.S. Centers for Disease Control and Prevention, last reviewed July 21, 2022, https://www.cdc.gov/chronicdisease/about/index.htm.

3   Wullianallur Raghupathi and Viju Raghupathi, "An Empirical Study of Chronic Diseases in the United States: A Visual Analytics Approach to Public Health," *International Journal of Environmental Research and Public Health* 15, no. 3 (March 2018): 431, https://doi.org/10.3390/ijerph15030431.

4   "Mental Health by the Numbers," National Alliance on Mental Illness, last modified April 2023, https://www.nami.org/mhstats.

5   "Facts about Suicide," U.S. Centers for Disease Control and Prevention, last reviewed May 8, 2023, https://www.cdc.gov/suicide/facts/index.html.

6   National Center for Health Statistics, "U.S. Overdose Deaths in 2021 Increased Half as Much as in 2020—but Are Still Up 15%," press release, May 11, 2022, https://www.cdc.gov/nchs/pressroom/nchs_press_releases/2022/202205.htm.

7   "Deaths from Excessive Alcohol Use in the United States," U.S. Centers for Disease Control and Prevention, last reviewed July 6, 2022, https://www.cdc.gov/alcohol/features/excessive-alcohol-deaths.html.

8   "NHE Fact Sheet," U.S. Centers for Medicare and Medicaid Services, last modified February 17, 2023, https://www.cms.gov/Research-Statistics-Data-and-Systems/Statistics-Trends-and-Reports/NationalHealthExpendData/NHE-Fact-Sheet.

9   Naykky Singh Ospina et al., "Eliciting the Patient's Agenda—Secondary Analysis of Recorded Clinical Encounters," *Journal of General Internal Medicine* 34, no. 1 (January 2019): 36–40, https://doi.org/10.1007/s11606-018-4540-5.

10 Marty Makary, *The Price We Pay: What Broke American Health Care—And How to Fix It* (New York: Bloomsbury Publishing, 2019).

11 James T. Boffetti, "Attorney General Formella [sic] Announces Up to $6 Billion National Settlement with Purdue Pharma and Sacklers; New Hampshire to Receive $46 Million If Agreement Approved," news release, March 3, 2022, New Hampshire Department of Justice, Office of the Attorney General, https://www.doj.nh.gov/news/2022/20220303-settlement-purdue-pharma-sacklers.htm.

12 "Understanding the Opioid Overdose Epidemic," U.S. Centers for Disease Control and Prevention, last reviewed June 1, 2022, https://www.cdc.gov/opioids/basics/epidemic.html.

13 Ming Tai-Seale, Thomas G. McGuire, and Weimin Zhang, "Time Allocation in Primary Care Office Visits," *Health Services Research* 42, no. 5 (October 2007): 1871–1894, https://doi.org/10.1111/j.1475-6773.2006.00689.x.

14 Misha Segal et al., "Medicare-Medicaid Eligible Beneficiaries and Potentially Avoidable Hospitalizations," *Medicare and Medicaid Research Review* 4, no. 1 (2014): E1–E10, http://dx.doi.org/10.5600/mmrr.004.01.b01

15 Vineet M. Arora et al., "Problems after Discharge and Understanding of Communication with their PCPs among Hospitalized Seniors: A Mixed Methods Study," *Journal of Hospital Medicine* 5, no. 7 (September 2010): 385–391, https://doi.org/10.1002/jhm.668.

16 Marilyn J. Field and Kathleen N. Lohr, eds., *Clinical Practice Guidelines: Directions for a New Program* (Washington, D.C.: National Academies Press, Institute of Medicine, 1990), 8, https://doi.org/10.17226/1626.

17 Roger L. Sur and Philipp Dahm, "History of Evidence-Based Medicine," *Indian Journal of Urology* 27, no. 4 (October–December 2011): 487–489, https://doi.org/10.4103/0970-1591.91438.

18 Dimitra Panteli et al., "Clinical Practice Guidelines as a Quality Strategy," in *Improving Healthcare Quality in Europe: Characteristics, Effectiveness and Implementation of Different Strategies*, Health Policy Series 53, eds. Reinhard Busse et al. (Copenhagen: European Observatory on Health Systems and Policies, 2019), 233–263, https://www.ncbi.nlm.nih.gov/books/NBK549283/.

19 K. Daniel Rose and Irving Rosow, "Physicians Who Kill Themselves," *Archives of General Psychiatry* 29, no. 6 (December 1973): 800–805, http://doi.org/10.1001/archpsyc.1973.04200060072011; Louise B. Andrew, "Physician Suicide," Medscape, last updated July 13, 2022, https://emedicine.medscape.com/article/806779-overview.

20 Eva S. Schernhammer and Graham A. Colditz, "Suicide Rates among Physicians: A Quantitative and Gender Assessment (Meta-Analysis)," *The American Journal of Psychiatry* 161, no. 12 (December 2004): 2295–2302, https://doi.org/10.1176/appi.ajp.161.12.2295; Dario M. Torre et al., "Suicide Compared to Other Causes of Mortality in Physicians," *Suicide and Life-Threatening Behavior* 35, no. 2 (April 2005): 146–153, https://doi.org/10.1521/suli.35.2.146.62878.

21 Samuel B. Harvey et al., "Mental Illness and Suicide among Physicians," *The Lancet* 398, no. 10303 (September 4, 2021): 920–930, https://doi.org/10.1016/S0140-6736(21)01596-8.

22 Dike Drummond, "Physician Burnout: Its Origin, Symptoms, and Five Main Causes," *Family Practice Management* 22, no. 5 (September/October 2015): 42–47, https://www.aafp.org/pubs/fpm/issues/2015/0900/p42.html.

23 Merritt Hawkins, *2018 Survey of America's Physicians: Practice Patterns and Perspectives* (Austin: The Physicians Foundation, 2018), 7–8, https://physiciansfoundation.org/wp-content/uploads/2018/09/physicians-survey-results-final-2018.pdf.

24 Karen Gilchrist, "Covid Has Made It Harder to Be a Health-Care Worker. Now, Many Are Thinking of Quitting," CNBC, last updated June 1, 2021, https://www.cnbc.com/2021/05/31/covid-is-driving-an-exodus-among-health-care-workers.html.

25 John Murphy, "Nearly Half of Doctors Are Rethinking Their Careers, Finds COVID-19 Survey," MDLinx, November 6, 2020, https://www.mdlinx.com/article/nearly-half-of-doctors-are-rethinking-their-careers-finds-covid-19-survey/32iphKz3vp3DlR3LuXO BkA.

26 Celli Horstman and Corinne Lewis, "How Primary Care Is Faring Two Years into the COVID-19 Pandemic," *To The Point* (blog), The Commonwealth Fund, February 23, 2022, https://doi.org/10.26099/zzvh-rb70.

27 Victoria Knight, "American Medical Students Less Likely to Choose to Become Primary Care Doctors," Kaiser Health News, July 3, 2019, https://khn.org/news/american-medical-students-less-likely-to-choose-to-become-primary-care-doctors/.

28 Chris Mazzolini and Logan Lutton, "Are Primary Care Physicians Underpaid? New Study Suggests the Answer Is Yes," *Medical Economics*, June 30, 2019, https://www.medicaleconomics.com/view/are-primary-care-physicians-underpaid-new-study-suggests-answer-yes.

29 John Torinus, Jr., *The Company that Solved Health Care: How Serigraph Dramatically Reduced Skyrocketing Costs while Providing Better Care, and How Every Company Can Do the Same* (Dallas: BenBella Books, 2010).

30 "Cost of Care: How Americans Have Paid for Healthcare throughout History," Arcadia Publishing, accessed May 8, 2023, https://www.arcadiapublishing.com/Navigation/Community/Arcadia-and-THP-Blog/August-2017/Cost-of-Care-How-Americans-Have-Paid-for-Healthca.

31 Siang Yong Tan and Yvonne Tatsumura, "Alexander Fleming (1881–1955): Discoverer of Penicillin," *Singapore Medical Journal* 56, no. 7 (2015): 366–367, https://doi.org/10.11622/smedj.2015105.

32 Daniel H. Robinson and Alexander H. Toledo, "Historical Development of Modern Anesthesia," *Journal of Investigative Surgery* 25, no. 3 (2012): 141–149, https://doi.org/10.3109/089 41939.2012.690328.

33 Thomas P. Duffy, "The Flexner Report—100 Years Later," *Yale Journal of Biology and Medicine* 84, no. 3 (September 2011): 269–276, https://www.ncbi.nlm.nih.gov/pmc/articles/PMC3178858/pdf/yjbm_84_3_269.pdf.

34 Barbra Mann Wall, "History of Hospitals," Penn Nursing, accessed March 16, 2023, https://www.nursing.upenn.edu/nhhc/nurses-institutions-caring/history-of-hospitals/.

35 "An Industry Pioneer," Blue Cross Blue Shield, accessed May 16, 2023, https://www.bcbs.com/about-us/industry-pioneer.

36 Marilyn J. Field and Harold T. Shapiro, eds., "Origins and Evolution of Employment-Based Health Benefits," chap. 2 in *Employment and Health Benefits: A Connection at Risk* (Washington, DC: National Academies Press, 1993), 49–86, https://doi.org/10.17226/2044.

37 Edward Berkowitz, "Medicare and Medicaid: The Past as Prologue," *Health Care Financing Review* 27, no. 2 (Winter 2005–2006): 11–23, https://pubmed.ncbi.nlm.nih.gov/17290633/.

38 Fred D. Ledley et al., "Profitability of Large Pharmaceutical Companies Compared with Other Large Public Companies," *JAMA* 323, no. 9 (March 3, 2020): 834–843, https://doi.org/10.1001/jama.2020.0442.

39 Melissa A. Thomasson, "From Sickness to Health: The Twentieth-Century Development of U.S. Health Insurance," *Exploration in Economic History* 39, no. 3 (July 2002): 233–253, https://doi.org/10.1006/exeh.2002.0788.

40 Arnold S. Relman, "The New Medical-Industrial Complex," *The New England Journal of Medicine* 303, no. 17 (October 23, 1980): 963–970, https://doi.org/10.1056/NEJM198010233031703.

41 Imani Telesford et al., "How Has U.S. Spending on Healthcare Changed over Time?," Peterson-KFF Health System Tracker, February 7, 2023, https://www.healthsystemtracker.org/chart-collection/u-s-spending-healthcare-changed-time/.

42 David Kotelchuck, ed., *Prognosis Negative: Crisis in the Health Care System* (New York: Vintage Books, 1976), 345–347.

43 Alain Enthoven, "The Rise and Fall of HMOs Shows How a Worthy Idea Went Wrong," *CommonWealth Magazine*, April 10, 2005, https://commonwealthmagazine.org/arts-and-culture/emthe-rise-and-fall-of-hmosm-shows-how-a-worthy-idea-went-wrong/.

44 "Preferred Provider Organization (PPO)," Healthcare.gov, accessed March 16, 2023, https://www.healthcare.gov/glossary/preferred-provider-organization-ppo/.

45 Michael E. Porter, "A Strategy for Health Care Reform—Toward a Value-Based System," *The New England Journal of Medicine* 361, no. 2 (July 2009): 109–112, https://doi.org/10.1056/NEJMp0904131.

46 Michael E. Porter, "What Is Value in Health Care?" *The New England Journal of Medicine* 363, no. 26 (December 2010): 2477–2481, https://doi.org/10.1056/NEJMp1011024.

47 "Quality Measures," U.S. Centers for Medicare and Medicaid Services, last modified April 14, 2022, https://www.cms.gov/Medicare/Quality-Initiatives-Patient-Assessment-Instruments/QualityMeasures.

48 "About the CMS Innovation Center," U.S. Centers for Medicare and Medicaid Services, last modified April 18, 2023, https://innovation.cms.gov/about.

49 "Accountable Care Organizations (ACOs): General Information," U.S. Centers for Medicare and Medicaid Services, last modified April 13, 2023, https://innovation.cms.gov/innovation-models/aco.

50 "Primary Care First Model Options," U.S. Centers for Medicare and Medicaid Services, last modified April 14, 2023, https://innovation.cms.gov/innovation-models/primary-care-first-model-options.

51 Yalda Jabbarpour et al., *Advanced Primary Care: A Key Contributor to Successful ACOs* (Washington, DC: Patient-Centered Primary Care Collaborative and Robert Graham Center, August 2018), 19–23, https://www.pcpcc.org/sites/default/files/resources/PCPCC%202018%20Evidence%20Report.pdf.

52 U.S. Centers for Medicare and Medicaid Services, "Affordable Care Act's Shared Savings Program Continues to Improve Quality of Care While Saving Medicare Money during the COVID-19 Pandemic," press release, August 25, 2021, https://www.cms.gov/newsroom/press-releases/affordable-care-acts-shared-savings-program-continues-improve-quality-care-while-saving-medicare.

53 "Hospital Readmissions Reduction Program (HRRP)," U.S. Centers for Medicare and Medicaid Services, last modified August 8, 2022, https://www.cms.gov/Medicare/Quality-Initiatives-Patient-Assessment-Instruments/Value-Based-Programs/HRRP/Hospital-Readmission-Reduction-Program.

54 Mabelle Regi Arole and Rajanikant Arole, *Jamkhed: A Comprehensive Rural Health Project* (New York: Macmillan, 1994).

55 Heather Landi, "Most Health Systems Still Base Doctors' Pay on Volume, Despite Push toward Value-Based Care: Study," Fierce Healthcare, January 28, 2022, https://www.fiercehealthcare.com/practices/most-health-systems-still-base-doctors-pay-volume-despite-push-towards-value-based-care.

56   "NHE Fact Sheet," U.S. Centers for Medicare and Medicaid Services, last modified February 17, 2023, https://www.cms.gov/Research-Statistics-Data-and-Systems/Statistics-Trends-and-Reports/NationalHealthExpendData/NHE-Fact-Sheet.

57   "The Spiritual Exercises," Ignatian Spirituality, accessed March 16, 2023, https://www.ignatianspirituality.com/ignatian-prayer/the-spiritual-exercises/.

58   James Gleick, *Chaos: Making a New Science* (New York: Viking Adult, 1987); Jack Cohen and Ian Stewart, *The Collapse of Chaos: Discovering Simplicity in a Complex World* (London: Penguin Books, 1994); Stuart Kauffman, *At Home in the Universe: The Search for the Laws of Self-Organization and Complexity* (New York: Oxford University Press, 1995).

59   Edda Klipp et al., *Systems Biology: A Textbook*, 2nd ed. (Weinheim, Germany: Wiley-VCH, 2016), xi–xii; Institute for Systems Biology, "What Is Systems Biology," ISBSceince.org, accessed March 16, 2023, https://isbscience.org/about/what-is-systems-biology/.

60   Albert-László Barabási, Natali Gulbahce, and Joseph Loscalzo, "Network Medicine: A Network-Based Approach to Human Disease," *Nature Reviews: Genetics* 12, no. 1 (2011): 56–68, https://doi.org/10.1038/nrg2918.

61   Massimo S. Fiandaca et al., "Systems Healthcare: A Holistic Paradigm for Tomorrow," *BMC Systems Biology* 11, no. 1 (2017): 142, https://doi.org/10.1186/s12918-017-0521-2.

62   Hiroaki Kitano, "Grand Challenges in Systems Physiology," *Frontiers in Physiology* 1 (2013): 3, https://doi.org/10.3389/fphys.2010.00003.

63   Leroy Hood, Rudi Balling, and Charles Auffray, "Revolutionizing Medicine in the 21st Century through Systems Approaches," *Biotechnology Journal* 7, no. 8 (August 2012): 992–1001, https://doi.org/10.1002/biot.201100306.

64   Mauricio Flores et al., "P4 Medicine: How Systems Medicine Will Transform the Healthcare Sector and Society," *Personalized Medicine* 10, no. 6 (2013): 565–576, https://doi.org/10.2217/pme.13.57.

65   Christopher J. Phillips, "Precision Medicine and Its Imprecise History," *Harvard Data Science Review* 2, no. 1 (Winter 2020), https://doi.org/10.1162/99608f92.3e85b56a.

66   "The Precision Medicine Initiative," The White House of President Barack Obama, accessed March 16, 2023, https://obamawhitehouse.archives.gov/precision-medicine.

67   Kalliopi Trachana et al., "Taking Systems Medicine to Heart," *Circulation Research* 122, no. 9 (2018): 1276–1289, https://doi.org/10.1161/CIRCRESAHA.117.310999.

68   American Heart Association editorial staff, "Lifestyle Changes for Heart Attack Prevention," American Heart Association, last reviewed July 31, 2015, https://www.heart.org/en/health-topics/heart-attack/life-after-a-heart-attack/lifestyle-changes-for-heart-attack-prevention.

69 National Diabetes Prevention Program, "Lifestyle Change Program Providers," U.S. Centers for Disease Control and Prevention, last reviewed December 27, 2022, https://www.cdc.gov/diabetes/prevention/program-providers.htm.

70 Kurt C. Stange, Robert L. Ferrer, and William L. Miller, "Making Sense of Health Care Transformation as Adaptive-Renewal Cycles," *Annals of Family Medicine* 7, no. 6 (November 2009): 484–487, https://doi.org/10.1370/afm.1032.

71 Susan E. Skochelak et al., eds., *Health Science Systems*, 2nd ed. (Amsterdam: Elsevier, 2021), ix.

72 Shelli R. Kesler, "Turner Syndrome," *Child and Adolescent Psychiatric Clinics of North America* 16, no. 3 (July 2007): 709–722, https://doi.org/10.1016/j.chc.2007.02.004.

73 Danielle Ligenza, "Sir William Osler, the 'Father of Modern Medicine,'" *Barton Blog*, Barton Associates, July 30, 2015, https://www.bartonassociates.com/blog/sir-william-osler-the-father-of-modern-medicine/.

74 Peter Sterling, *What Is Health?: Allostasis and the Evolution of Human Design* (Cambridge, MA: The MIT Press, 2020), 154.

75 Katsutaro Morino, Kitt Falk Petersen, and Gerald I. Shulman, "Molecular Mechanisms of Insulin Resistance in Humans and Their Potential Links with Mitochondrial Dysfunction," *Diabetes* 55, Supplement 2 (December 2006): S9–S15, https://doi.org/10.2337/db06-S002.

76 Jonathan C. Cohen et al., "Sequence Variations in PCSK9, Low LDL, and Protection against Coronary Heart Disease," *The New England Journal of Medicine* 354, no. 12 (March 2006): 1264–1272, https://doi.org/10.1056/NEJMoa054013.

77 Chelsea Toledo and Kirstie Saltsman, "Genetics by the Numbers," *Inside Life Science* (blog), National Institute of General Medical Sciences, June 12, 2012, https://nigms.nih.gov/education/Inside-Life-Science/Pages/Genetics-by-the-Numbers.aspx.

78 Majesta O'Bleness et al., "Evolution of Genetic and Genomic Features Unique to the Human Lineage," *Nature Reviews: Genetics* 13, no. 12 (December 2012): 853–866, https://doi.org/10.1038/nrg3336.

79 Kevin Esoh and Ambroise Wonkam, "Evolutionary History of Sickle-Cell Mutation: Implications for Global Genetic Medicine," *Human Molecular Genetics* 30, no. R1 (March 2021): R119–R128, https://doi.org/10.1093/hmg/ddab004.

80 George Davey Smith et al., "Lactase Persistence-Related Genetic Variant: Population Substructure and Health Outcomes," *European Journal of Human Genetics* 17 (2009): 357–367, https://doi.org/10.1038/ejhg.2008.156.

81 Misganaw Asmamaw and Belay Zawdie, "Mechanism and Applications of CRISPR/Cas-9-Mediated Genome Editing," *Biologics* 2021, no. 15 (2021): 353–361, https://doi.org/10.2147/BTT.S326422.

82 Marten Scheffer, Critical Transitions in Nature and Society (Princeton, NJ: Princeton University Press, 2009); Ugo Bardi, *Before the Collapse: A Guide to the Other Side of Growth* (Cham, Switzerland: Springer, 2020), https://doi.org/10.1007/978-3-030-29038-2.

83 Marten Scheffer et al., "Early-Warning Signals for Critical Transitions," *Nature* 461, no. 7260 (2009): 53–59, https://doi.org/10.1038/nature08227.

84 National Center for Chronic Disease Prevention and Health Promotion, Division of Population Health, "Osteoarthritis (OA)," U.S. Centers for Disease Control and Prevention, last reviewed July 27, 2020, https://www.cdc.gov/arthritis/basics/osteoarthritis.htm.

85 "Plastic Surgeons in the US—Market Size 2005–2028," IBIS World, last updated February 24, 2023,https://www.ibisworld.com/industry-statistics/market-size/plastic-surgeons-united-states/.

86 Martha Hotz Vitaterna, Joseph S. Takahashi, and Fred W. Turek, "Overview of Circadian Rhythms," *Alcohol Research and Health* 25, no. 2 (2001): 85–93, https://pubmed.ncbi.nlm.nih.gov/11584554/.

87 U.S. Centers for Disease Control and Prevention, *Picture of America: Heart-Related Illness* (Washington, DC: U.S. Centers for Disease Control and Prevention, accessed March 16, 2023), 1, https://www.cdc.gov/pictureofamerica/pdfs/picture_of_america_heat-related_illness.pdf.

88 "QuickStats: Number of Hypothermia-Related Deaths by Sex—National Vital Statistics System, United States, 1999–2011," *Morbidity and Mortality Weekly Report* 61, no. 51 (January 4, 2013): 1050, https://www.cdc.gov/mmwr/preview/mmwrhtml/mm6151a6.htm.

89 "Harms of Cigarette Smoking and Health Benefits of Quitting," National Cancer Institute, last reviewed December 19, 2017, https://www.cancer.gov/about-cancer/causes-prevention/risk/tobacco/cessation-fact-sheet.

90 Claudia Campanale et al., "A Detailed Review Study on Potential Effects of Microplastics and Additives of Concern on Human Health," *International Journal of Environmental Research and Public Health* 17, no. 4 (February 2020): 1212, https://doi.org/10.3390/ijerph17041212.

91 Lien Ai Pham-Huy, Hua He, and Chuong Pham-Huy, "Free Radicals, Antioxidants in Disease and Health," *International Journal of Biomedical Science* 4, no. 2 (June 2008): 89–96, https://pubmed.ncbi.nlm.nih.gov/23675073/.

92 Jack A. Gilbert et al., "Current Understanding of the Human Microbiome," *Nature Medicine* 24, no. 4 (April 2018): 392–400, https://doi.org/10.1038/nm.4517.

93 Yong Fan and Oluf Pedersen, "Gut Microbiota in Human Metabolic Health and Disease," *Nature Reviews Microbiology* 19, no. 1 (2021): 55–71, https://doi.org/10.1038/s41579-020-0433-9.

94 Paul Webster, "Antibiotic Overprescribing a Growing Problem," *Canadian Medical Association Journal* 189, no. 5 (February 2017): E222, https://doi.org/10.1503/cmaj.1095383.

95 Longfei Yang et al., "The Effects of Psychological Stress on Depression," *Current Neuropharmacology* 13, no. 4 (2015): 494–504, https://doi.org/10.2174/1570159X1304150831150507.

96 Firdaus S. Dhabhar, "The Short-Term Stress Response—Mother Nature's Mechanism for Enhancing Protection and Performance under Conditions of Threat, Challenge, and Opportunity," *Frontiers in Neuroendocrinology* 49 (April 2018): 175–192, https://doi.org/10.1016/j.yfrne.2018.03.004.

97 Mayo Clinic Staff, "Chronic Stress Puts Your Health at Risk," Mayo Clinic, July 8, 2021, https://www.mayoclinic.org/healthy-lifestyle/stress-management/in-depth/stress/art-20046037.

98 Sonya B. Norman and Shira Maguen, "PTSD: National Center for PTSD," U.S. Department of Veterans Affairs, last modified July 26, 2021, https://www.ptsd.va.gov/professional/treat/cooccurring/moral_injury.asp.

99 Brett T. Litz et al., "Moral Injury and Moral Repair in War Veterans: A Preliminary Model and Intervention Strategy," *Clinical Psychology Review* 29, no. 8 (December 2009): 695–706, https://doi.org/10.1016/j.cpr.2009.07.003.

100 James Krieger and Donna L. Higgins, "Housing and Health: Time Again for Public Health Action," *American Journal of Public Health* 92, no. 5 (May 2002): 758–768, https://doi.org/10.2105/AJPH.92.5.758.

101 B. Ronan O'Driscoll, Linda C. Hopkinson, and David W. Denning, "Mold Sensitization Is Common amongst Patients with Severe Asthma Requiring Multiple Hospital Admissions," *BMC Pulmonary Medicine* 5, no. 4 (2005), https://doi.org/10.1186/1471-2466-5-4.

102 Tomaz Velnar, T. Bailey, and V. Smrkolj, "The Wound Healing Process: An Overview of the Cellular and Molecular Mechanisms," *Journal of International Medical Research* 37, no. 5 (September/October 2009): 1528–1542, https://doi.org/10.1177/147323000903700531.

103 A. Agrawal et al., "The Genetics of Addiction—A Translational Perspective," *Translational Psychiatry* 2, no. 7 (July 2012): e140, https://doi.org/10.1038/tp.2012.54.

104 Tammy Saah, "The Evolutionary Origins and Significance of Drug Addiction," *Harm Reduction Journal* 2 (2005): 8, https://doi.org/10.1186/1477-7517-2-8.

105 Anna Lembke, *Dopamine Nation: Finding Balance in the Age of Indulgence* (New York: Dutton, 2021).

106 "Keep on Your Feet—Preventing Older Adult Falls," Injury Prevention and Control, U.S. Centers for Disease Control and Prevention, last reviewed March 24, 2023, https://www.cdc.gov/injury/features/older-adult-falls/index.html.

107 Linda P. Fried et al., "Frailty in Older Adults: Evidence for a Phenotype," *The Journals of Gerontology: Series A* 56, no. 3 (March 2001): M146–M157, https://doi.org/10.1093/gerona/56.3.M146.

108 Linda P. Fried et al., "The Physical Frailty Syndrome as a Transition from Homeostatic Symphony to Cacophony," *Nature Aging* 1, no. 1 (January 2021): 36–46, https://doi.org/10.1038/s43587-020-00017-z.

109 Linda P. Fried et al., "Nonlinear Multisystem Physiological Dysregulation Associated with Frailty in Older Women: Implications for Etiology and Treatment," *The Journals of Gerontology: Series A* 64A, no. 10 (October 2009): 1049–1057, https://doi.org/10.1093/gerona/glp076.

110 James F. Fries, "The Compression of Morbidity," *The Milbank Quarterly* 83, no. 4 (December 2005): 801–823, https://doi.org/10.1111/j.1468-0009.2005.00401.x.

111 Freda Kreier, "Wide-Ranging Genetic Study of Severe COVID Finds Common Risk Factors," *Nature*, March 10, 2022, https://doi.org/10.1038/d41586-022-00677-4; SeyedAhmad SeyedAlinaghi et al., "Minimum Infective Dose of Severe Acute Respiratory Syndrome Coronavirus 2 Based on the Current Evidence: A Systematic Review," *SAGE Open Medicine* 10 (January–December 2022), https://doi.org/10.1177/20503121221115053; "People with Certain Medical Conditions," Your Health, COVID-19, U.S. Centers for Disease Control and Prevention, last modified February 10, 2023, https://www.cdc.gov/coronavirus/2019-ncov/need-extra-precautions/people-with-medical-conditions.html.

112 Peter Sterling, *What Is Health?: Allostasis and the Evolution of Human Design* (Cambridge, MA: The MIT Press, 2020).

113 William S. Queale and Linda P. Fried, "Advanced Activities of Daily Living in Healthy Older Women," paper presented at the Society of General Internal Medicine Annual Conference, San Francisco, CA, April 1999.

114 Doowon Lee et al., "Effects of Individualized Low-Intensity Exercise and Its Duration on Recovery Ability in Adults," *Healthcare* 9, no. 3 (2021): 249, https://doi.org/10.3390/healthcare9030249.

115 Jonathan M. Memme et al., "Exercise and Mitochondrial Health," *The Journal of Physiology* 599, no. 3 (February 2021): 803–817, https://doi.org/10.1113/JP278853.

116 Julia Szendroedi, Esther Phielix, and Michael Roden, "The Role of Mitochondria in Insulin Resistance and Type 2 Diabetes Mellitus," *Nature Reviews: Endocrinology* 8, no. 2 (2012): 92–103, https://doi.org/10.1038/nrendo.2011.138.

117 Karolina Talar et al., "Benefits of Resistance Training in Early and Late Stages of Frailty and Sarcopenia: A Systematic Review and Meta-Analysis of Randomized Controlled Studies," *Journal of Clinical Medicine* 10, no. 8 (April 2021): 1630, https://doi.org/10.3390/jcm10081630.

118 Wayne L. Westcott, "Resistance Training Is Medicine: Effects of Strength Training on Health," *Current Sports Medicine Reports* 11, no. 4 (July/August 2012): 209–216, https://doi.org/10.1249/JSR.0b013e31825dabb8.

119 Robert A. Saxton and David M. Sabatini, "mTOR Signaling in Growth, Metabolism, and Disease," *Cell* 168, no. 6 (March 2017): 960–976, https://doi.org/10.1016/j.cell.2017.02.004.

120 Muhammed Mustafa Atakan et al., "Evidence-Based Effects of High-Intensity Interval Training on Exercise Capacity and Health: A Review with Historical Perspective," *International Journal of Environmental Research and Public Health* 18, no. 13 (July 2021): 7201, https://doi.org/10.3390/ijerph18137201.

121 Reuben L. Smith et al., "Metabolic Flexibility as an Adaptation to Energy Resources and Requirements in Health and Disease," *Endocrine Reviews* 39, no. 4 (August 2018): 489–517, https://doi.org/10.1210/er.2017-00211.

122 Laura Mandolesi et al., "Effects of Physical Exercise on Cognitive Functioning and Wellbeing: Biological and Psychological Benefits," *Frontiers in Psychology* 9 (2018): 509, https://doi.org/10.3389/fpsyg.2018.00509.

123 C. B. Hall et al., "Cognitive Activities Delay Onset of Memory Decline in Persons Who Develop Dementia," *Neurology* 73, no. 5 (August 2009): 356–361, https://doi.org/10.1212/WNL.0b013e3181b04ae3.

124 Esther G. A. Karssemeijer et al., "Positive Effects of Combined Cognitive and Physical Exercise Training on Cognitive Function in Older Adults with Mild Cognitive Impairment or Dementia: A Meta-Analysis," *Aging Research Reviews* 40 (November 2017): 75–83, https://doi.org/10.1016/j.arr.2017.09.003.

125 Fatih Ozbay et al., "Social Support and Resilience to Stress: From Neurobiology to Clinical Practice," *Psychiatry* 4, no. 5 (May 2007): 35–40, https://pubmed.ncbi.nlm.nih.gov/20806028/.

126 Kathleen M. MacQueen et al., "What Is Community? An Evidence-Based Definition for Participatory Public Health," *American Journal of Public Health* 91, no. 12 (December 2001): 1929–1938, https://doi.org/10.2105/AJPH.91.12.1929.

127 Joanne Slavin and Justin Carlson, "Carbohydrates," *Advances in Nutrition* 5, no. 6 (November 2014): 760–761, https://doi.org/10.3945/an.114.006163.

128 James W. Anderson et al., "Health Benefits of Dietary Fiber," *Nutrition Reviews* 67, no. 4 (April 2009): 188–205, https://doi.org/10.1111/j.1753-4887.2009.00189.x.

129 Asmaa S. Abdelhamid et al., "Polyunsaturated Fatty Acids for the Primary and Secondary Prevention of Cardiovascular Disease," *Cochrane Database of Systematic Reviews* 2018, no. 11 (November 2018), https://doi.org/10.1002/14651858.CD012345.pub3.

130 Sally Chiu, Paul T. Williams, and Ronald M. Krauss, "Effects of a Very High Saturated Fat Diet on LDL Particles in Adults with Atherogenic Dyslipidemia: A Randomized Controlled Trial," *PLoS ONE* 12, no. 2 (2017): e0170664, https://doi.org/10.1371/journal.pone.0170664.

131 Donald K. Layman et al., "Defining Meal Requirements for Protein to Optimize Metabolic Roles of Amino Acids," *The American Journal of Clinical Nutrition* 101, no. 6 (June 2015): 1330S–1338S, https://doi.org/10.3945/ajcn.114.084053.

132   Malcolm Watford and Guoyao Wu, "Protein," *Advances in Nutrition* 9, no. 5 (September 2018): 651–653, https://doi.org/10.1093/advances/nmy027.

133   A. Shenkin, "Micronutrients in Health and Disease," *Postgraduate Medical Journal* 82, no. 971 (September 2006): 559–567, https://doi.org/10.1136/pgmj.2006.047670.

134   Yiren Wang and Ruilin Wu, "The Effect of Fasting on Human Metabolism and Psychological Health," *Disease Markers* 2022 (January 2022): 5653739, https://doi.org/10.1155/2022/5653739.

135   Daniela Omodei and Luigi Fontana, "Calorie Restriction and Prevention of Age-Associated Chronic Disease," *FEBS Letters* 585, no. 11 (June 6, 2011): 1537–1542, https://doi.org/10.1016/j.febslet.2011.03.015.

136   Xiaojiao Zheng, Shouli Wang, and Wei Jia, "Calorie Restriction and Its Impact on Gut Microbial Composition and Global Metabolism," *Frontiers of Medicine* 12, no. 6 (December 2018): 634–644, https://doi.org/10.1007/s11684-018-0670-8.

137   Noboru Mizushima and Masaaki Komatsu, "Autophagy: Renovation of Cells and Tissues," *Cell* 147, no. 4 (November 11, 2011): 728–741, https://doi.org/10.1016/j.cell.2011.10.026.

138   Fiona Limanaqi et al., "Autophagy-Based Hypothesis on the Role of Brain Catecholamine Response during Stress," *Frontiers in Psychiatry* 11 (September 17, 2020): 569248, https://doi.org/10.3389/fpsyt.2020.569248.

139   Matthew Walker, *Why We Sleep: Unlocking the Power of Sleep and Dreams* (New York: Scribner, 2017), 107–192.

140   Mark E. Vogel et al., "Integration of Behavioral Health and Primary Care: Current Knowledge and Future Directions," *Journal of Behavioral Medicine* 40, no. 1 (2017): 69–84, https://doi.org/10.1007/s10865-016-9798-7.

141   Phillip Miller, *2017 Survey of Physician Appointment Wait Times and Medicare and Medicaid Acceptance Rates* (Dallas: Merritt Hawkins, 2017), 20–29, https://www.aristamd.com/wp-content/uploads/2018/11/mha2017waittimesurveyPDF-1.pdf.

142   Emily Barson and Russ Latino, "Here's How to Solve the Looming Shortage of Doctors: Nurse Practitioners," *USA Today*, February 10, 2020, https://www.usatoday.com/story/opinion/2020/02/10/nurse-practitioners-best-option-solve-u-s-shortage-doctors-column/4627268002/.

143   Lisa Schottenfeld et al., *Creating Patient-Centered Team-Based Primary Care*, white paper, AHRQ Pub. No. 16-0002-EF (Rockville, MD: Agency for Healthcare Research and Quality, March 2016), https://www.ahrq.gov/sites/default/files/wysiwyg/ncepcr/tools/PCMH/creating-patient-centered-team-based-primary-care-white-paper.pdf.

144   Esther M. Friedman and Patricia K. Tong, *A Framework for Integrating Family Caregivers into the Health Care Team* (Santa Monica: RAND Corporation, 2020), 1, https://www.rand.org/pubs/research_reports/RRA105-1.html.

145 Peter O'Meara et al., "Community Paramedicine Model of Care: An Observational, Ethnographic Case Study," *BMC Health Services Research* 16 (2015): 39, https://doi.org/10.1186/s12913-016-1282-0.

146 Gale M. Lucas et al., "It's Only a Computer: Virtual Humans Increase Willingness to Disclose," *Computers in Human Behavior* 37 (August 2014): 94–100, https://doi.org/10.1016/j.chb.2014.04.043.

147 J. Hunter Young et al., "How Algorithms Could Improve Primary Care," *Harvard Business Review*, May 6, 2022, https://hbr.org/2022/05/how-algorithms-could-improve-primary-care.

148 NCI Staff, "Liquid Biopsy: Using DNA in Blood to Detect, Track, and Treat Cancer," *Cancer Currents Blog*, National Cancer Institute, November 8, 2017, https://www.cancer.gov/news-events/cancer-currents-blog/2017/liquid-biopsy-detects-treats-cancer.

149 Joo Heung Yoon et al., "Prediction of Hypotension Events with Physiologic Vital Sign Signatures in the Intensive Care Unit," *Critical Care* 24, no. 1 (December 2020): 661, https://doi.org/10.1186/s13054-020-03379-3.

150 Evan D. Muse et al., "Toward a Smart Medical Home," *The Lancet* 389, no. 10067 (January 28, 2017): 358, https://doi.org/10.1016/S0140-6736(17)30154-X.

151 U.S. Food and Drug Administration, "Precision Medicine," last modified September 27, 2018, https://www.fda.gov/medical-devices/in-vitro-diagnostics/precision-medicine.

152 Shabbir Ahmed et al, "Pharmacogenomics of Drug Metabolizing Enzymes and Transporters: Relevance to Precision Medicine," *Genomics, Proteomics and Bioinformatics* 14, no. 5 (October 2016): 298–313, https://doi.org/10.1016/j.gpb.2016.03.008.

153 Nelly N. Miteva-Marcheva et al., "Application of Pharmacogenetics in Oncology," *Biomarker Research* 8, no. 32 (2020), https://doi.org/10.1186/s40364-020-00213-4.

154 Vini Vijayan et al., "Review of Wearable Devices and Data Collection Considerations for Connected Health," *Sensors* 21, no. 16 (August 2021): 5589, https://doi.org/10.3390/s21165589.

155 Juliane R. Sempionatto et al., "Wearable Chemical Sensors for Biomarker Discovery in the Omics Era," *Nature Reviews: Chemistry* 6, no. 12 (2022): 899–915, https://doi.org/10.1038/s41570-022-00439-w.

156 J. Masison et al., "A Modular Computational Framework for Medical Digital Twins," *Proceedings of the National Academy of Sciences of the United States* 118, no. 20 (May 2021): e2024287118, https://doi.org/10.1073/pnas.2024287118.

157 Trisha Greenhalgh, "Intuition and Evidence—Uneasy Bedfellows?," *British Journal of General Practice* 52, no. 478 (May 2002): 395–400, https://www.ncbi.nlm.nih.gov/pmc/articles/PMC1314297/.

158 Trisha Torrey, "Differences between Primary, Secondary, Tertiary, and Quaternary Care," Verywell Health, last updated October 2, 2022, https://www.verywellhealth.com/primary-secondary-tertiary-and-quaternary-care-2615354.

159 Linda McCauley et al., eds., *Implementing High-Quality Primary Care: Rebuilding the Foundation of Health Care* (Washington, DC: National Academies Press, 2021), https://doi.org/10.17226/25983.

160 Vishal S. Arora and Sachin H. Jain, "What US Medicine Needs to Do to Finally Embrace Capitation," *Health Affairs Blog, Health Affairs Forefront*, November 3, 2020, https://doi.org/10.1377/forefront.20201029.440795.

161 "ACO REACH," U.S. Centers for Medicare and Medicaid Services, last modified March 24, 2023, https://innovation.cms.gov/innovation-models/aco-reach.

162 James M. Daniel, Jr., "Risk-Bearing Entities and Risk-Based Contracting," Hancock Daniel, accessed March 16, 2023, https://hancockdaniel.com/practice-areas/all-areas/healthcare/risk-bearing-entities/.

163 "Strategic Direction," U.S. Centers for Medicare and Medicaid Services, last modified April 18, 2023, https://innovation.cms.gov/strategic-direction.

164 Angelica Peebles, "Medicine's Worst-Paying Specialty Is Luring Billions from Wall Street," *Bloomberg*, February 10, 2022, https://www.bloomberg.com/news/features/2022-02-10/primary-care-health-investors-bet-billions-on-medicine-s-worst-paying-specialty?leadSource=uverify%20wall.

165 Ryan Crowley, Omar Atiq, and David Hilden, "Financial Profit in Medicine: A Position Paper from the American College of Physicians," *Annals of Internal Medicine* 174, no. 10 (October 2021): 1447–1449, https://doi.org/10.7326/M21-1178.

166 Yalda Jabbarpour et al., *Investing in Primary Care: A State-Level Analysis* (Washington, D.C.: Patient-Centered Primary Care Collaborative and the Robert Graham Center, July 2019), 5, https://www.graham-center.org/content/dam/rgc/documents/publications-reports/reports/Investing-Primary-Care-State-Level-PCMH-Report.pdf.

167 Patient-Centered Primary Care Collaborative, "Spending for Primary Care," August 2018, https://www.pcpcc.org/sites/default/files/resources/PCPCC%20Fact%20Sheet%20PC%20Spend%20Aug%202018.pdf.

168 Russell S. Phillips, "Investment in Primary Care Is Needed to Achieve the Triple Aim," *Health Affairs Blog, Health Affairs Forefront*, May 10, 2017, https://doi.org/10.1377/forefront.20170510.060008.

169 Mark McClellan et al., "Health Care Payers COVID-19 Impact Assessment: Lessons Learned and Compelling Needs," *NAM Perspectives* 2021 (May 17, 2021), https://doi.org/10.31478/202105a.

170 Association of American Medical Colleges, "New Report Confirms Growing Shortage of Primary Care Physicians," Primary Care Collaborative, July 10, 2020, https://www.pcpcc. org/2020/07/10/new-report-confirms-growing-shortage-primary-care-physicians.

171 "ChangeMedEd Initiative," American Medical Association, accessed March 16, 2023, https:// www.ama-assn.org/education/accelerating-change-medical-education.

172 Todd Shryock, "Hospitals Continue to Struggle with Margins as Costs Rise," *Medical Economics*, October 17, 2022, https://www.medicaleconomics.com/view/ hospitals-continue-to-struggle-with-margins-as-costs-rise.

173 Michael L. O'Dell, "What Is a Patient-Centered Medical Home?," *Missouri Medicine* 113, no. 4 (July–August 2016): 301–304, https://pubmed.ncbi.nlm.nih.gov/30228482/.

174 Jeff Tollefson, "Climate Change Is Hitting the Planet Faster than Scientists Originally Thought," *Nature*, February 28, 2022, https://doi.org/10.1038/d41586-022-00585-7.

175 Intergovernmental Panel on Climate Change, "Summary for Policymakers," In *The Ocean and Cryosphere in a Changing Climate: Special Report of the Intergovernmental Panel on Climate Change*, eds. Hans-Otto Pörtner et al. (Cambridge, UK: Cambridge University Press, 2022), 3–36, https://doi.org/10.1017/9781009157964.001.

176 Crescenti Y. Dakubo, "Exploring the Linkages Between Ecosystems and Human Health," In *Ecosystems and Human Health* (New York: Springer, 2010), 3–19, https://doi. org/10.1007/978-1-4419-0206-1_1.

177 Olivia Solon, "Elon Musk: We Must Colonise Mars to Preserve Our Species in a Third World War," *The Guardian*, March 11, 2018, https://www.theguardian.com/technology/2018/mar/11/ elon-musk-colonise-mars-third-world-war.

178 Mark Shelhamer "Why Send Humans into Space? Science and Non-Science Motivations for Human Space Flight," *Space Policy* 42 (November 2017): 37–40, https://doi.org/10.1016/j. spacepol.2017.10.001.

179 NASA, *NASA's Plan for Sustained Lunar Exploration and Development* (Washington, DC: NASA, 2019), 8–11, https://www.nasa.gov/sites/default/files/atoms/files/a_sustained_lunar_ presence_nspc_report4220final.pdf; Brian Dunbar, "Artemis," NASA, accessed March 16, 2023, https://www.nasa.gov/specials/artemis/.

180 "Communications," Mars 2020 Mission Perseverance Rover, NASA, accessed March 16, 2023, https://mars.nasa.gov/mars2020/spacecraft/rover/communications/.

Made in the USA
Middletown, DE
17 December 2023

46022559R00168